RENEWALS: 691-4574

DATE DUE

JUL 1 4			
APR 1 8			
APR 2 9			

Demco, Inc. 38-293

MEDICAL STEWARDSHIP

M. *Oliver Kepler*

MEDICAL STEWARDSHIP
Fulfilling the Hippocratic Legacy

Foreword by Joseph Fletcher

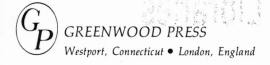

GP GREENWOOD PRESS
Westport, Connecticut • London, England

Library of Congress Cataloging in Publication Data

Kepler, Milton Oliver, 1920-
    Medical stewardship.

    Bibliography: p.
    Includes indexes.
    1. Medical ethics. I. Title. [DNLM: 1. Ethics,
Medical. W 50 K38m]
R724.K45   174'.2   80-25457
ISBN 0-313-22489-7 (lib. bdg.)

Library of Congress Catalog Card Number: 80-25457
ISBN: 0-313-22489-7

First published in 1981

Greenwood Press
A division of Congressional Information Service, Inc.
88 Post Road West
Westport, Connecticut 06881

Printed in the United States of America

10 9 8 7 6 5 4 3 2 1

This book is affectionately
dedicated to my parents, who
helped make it possible and
to my wife, Georgia, some
of whose ancestors started
it all.

How are we constituted by nature? To be free, to be noble, to be modest . . . and to subordinate pleasure to the ends for which Nature designed us, as a handmaid and a minister, in order to call forth our activity, in order to keep us constant to the path prescribed by Nature. *Epictetus*

CONTENTS

Foreword by Joseph Fletcher   xi

Preface   xiii

Chapter 1   Ancient Sources   3

Chapter 2   The Meaning of the Professional Person   16

Chapter 3   Forging an Ethical Device   22

Chapter 4   The Ethics of Medical Organization   24

Chapter 5   Marketplace Medicine and
            Patient Exploitation   45

Chapter 6   The Ethics of Professional Competence   53

Chapter 7   Some Underutilized Roles of the Physician   70

Chapter 8   The Ethics of Health-Care Provision:
            Responsible Medical Stewardship   102

Chapter 9   Experimentation On Humans and
            Patients' Rights   135

Chapter 10 Medicines Out of the Earth   146

Chapter 11 Philia Among Health Professionals   158

Chapter 12 Can the Medical Educators Learn?   178

Chapter 13 Toward an Ordered Whole   209

Appendix A American Hospital Association:
            A Patient's Bill of Rights   223

Appendix B	American Medical Association: Principles of Medical Ethics Version of 1957	227
Appendix C	American Medical Association: Principles of Medical Ethics Revision of 1980	231
Appendix D	California Natural Death Act Chapter 3.9	233
Appendix E	Concern for Dying: A Living Will	241
Appendix F	World Medical Association: Declaration of Geneva	243
Appendix G	World Medical Association: Declaration of Helsinki	245
Appendix H	Van Renssalaer Potter: A Bioethical Creed for Individuals	249
Notes		251
Bibliography		267
Author Index		271
Subject Index		273

FOREWORD

Joseph Fletcher

A mind and spirit able to embrace both the scientific speculations of sociobiology and the merits of the natural law tradition are rare. That breadth is Oliver Kepler's. It is this that accounts for his highly original examination of modern medicine and its ethics. Not often do we have a book which is critical without being cranky.

The inquiring reader will be frustrated if he comes to this book looking for still more doctor-baiting or another harangue about the "nemesis" of medicine. Doctor Kepler practices what he preaches; his words are where his action is. The perceptions he spells out for us are born of down-to-earth clinical experience, which nonetheless has never in the least dampened his will to ask good questions and to chase down good answers. He is a physician, yes, but most triumphantly a humanist.

It has always seemed to me that a good physician is one who understands the ambivalence of his art. Doctor Kepler's medical meditation perceives the two sides of *pharmakon* in a mature way; in Hippocrates's day the Greeks used the word to mean both medicine and poison. Medicine can cause trouble as well as relieve it, and sometimes the trouble goes with the relief—or even expedites it.

The Greeks also understood, just as Oliver Kepler does, that the essence of tragedy lies in the conflict or tension between one good and another. The conflict of good and evil is mere melodrama; it calls for none of the in-depth reflection that this book offers.

Someone once said that ethics is like breathing; we practice it all the time and have to. But few if any of the works on medical ethics nowadays attempt to put it in the historical, philosophical, and religious context that Doctor Kepler constructs—and constructs, I should say, without resorting to a dogmatic approach or hidden agenda. He does not, for example, play word games with terms such as "holistic medicine." These concepts come and go; what is sound in them is not new, and what is new is not sound.

Furthermore, what he has written is not just another casebook of the various problems of conscience that plague clinical medicine. I do not mean to downgrade the importance of normative ethics in medicine, but the fact is that Oliver Kepler has reached a greater depth. What he offers us, after many years of meditation, is a strikingly independent treatise of the "met-ethics" of medicine. It is this that gives his book its urbane as well as its humane dimension.

The author has also properly emphasized some underutilized roles of the physician; those of priest, comforter, advocate, and steward are often as important as the strictly medical one.

In times past physicians were perceived as Good Men, in Aristotle's sense of a good man as distinguished from a "good fellow." Their goodness was (1) sapient, they had special knowledge and skill; (2) moral, it was assumed they were concerned for their patients' interests first of all; and (3) charismatic, they were figures of grace and vocation.

This image has been weakened in all but the first respect, the sapient. If his message is understood, Oliver Kepler's book surely will go a long way toward redeeming the blurred parts of the image. I venture to adumbrate his message: physicians and their patients can and must think as well as know and build their visions as well as their data banks.

PREFACE

"Ethics?" grumbled a dental acquaintance of mine, "hell, you docs don't know what ethics is. We dentists really have ethics." Being curious, I pursued his remarks and found that the source of his annoyance was the number of restrictions placed on him by his local dental association. For instance, there was a prohibition against advertising and solicitation of patients, and a limit on the height of the letters on his office door and in the Yellow Pages. These and similar restrictions represented ethics to him, and apparently many physicians agree.

I must take a moment to clarify certain terms that will be used throughout this book. The terms "medical ethics" and "professional ethics" are often interchanged to mean restrictions or rules similar to the above and are commonly written up as "codes of ethics." Such restrictions on conduct are more properly called professional etiquette or custom. Similarly, "ethics" and "morals" are commonly interchanged but should not be. True ethics should involve principles rather than rigid codes and are relatively timeless. Morals, by distinction, are influenced by custom and differ with the times, the ethnic group, the location, and other factors. Ethics involves the individual or group in a demanding way, requiring reflection and decision as to how to act or refrain from acting.

This book is not concerned with medical ethics or etiquette in the narrow sense but rather the true ethics of health care. However, as a convention throughout this book I shall use the term "medical ethics" to mean the ethics of health care in the broad sense; the ethics involving health-care professionals in their daily activities. Such medical ethics determines much of the conduct between health-care professionals and those whom they serve.

Prior to entering medical school, I had many of the same misconceptions about what constituted medical ethics as my dental friend, and I found little in my formal education to alter my erroneous notions. Courses or other activities devoted to ethics were virtually unknown in the medical schools of my time, and I was entrapped in what has been called the "lock-step" of the then standardized medical curriculum. Electives were a rarity and offered only in basic or clinical medical science. This was the situation which largely prevailed for 50 years after the epochal Flexner report of 1911 which examined and reported on the status of medical education in this country.

However, I also went to medical school with another notion that I have retained and nurtured, and this basically is that the physician should be a very special person in a very special calling; similar to the type of person and calling visualized for a clergyman.

As my professional training progressed, I became more perplexed when my concepts were neither reinforced nor were my misconceptions corrected. Rather, I heard admonitions about what the successful physician must do to gain and keep patients. To be sure, I did encounter good and kind physicians in my training who did seem to have those special qualities I visualized as necessary for optimal patient care. But medical training was a mixed bag of role models with no one to indicate which type was desirable. I encountered little information on medical ethics except for the pre-1957 booklet *Code of Ethics* produced by the American Medical Association (AMA), and this was something of a disappointment since it spelled out a number of "dos" and "don'ts" rather than establishing ethical principles.

After a number of years of general medical practice I still had found little to guide me in certain situations. For example, should the physician always tell the truth to a patient? Should abortion be legalized? What were the rights of patients? What about prolonging life in a helpless case? In addition, more general medical-social issues such as socialized medicine, the right to medical care, and the obligations, if any, to serve the indigent, were all nagging me to take some stand.

Ultimately, I realized that I had to learn more if I wanted a more fulfilling practice of medicine. I had always had an interest in being a clergyman, but I had finally abandoned this inclination in favor of medicine. Why not look to the disciplines of religion and philosophy for help? After considerable soul-searching and a lot of dialog with some good people who shared some of my concerns, I decided I needed to go back to the old ivory tower. Some fourteen years after graduation from medical school I found myself going through the perils of academic registration and choosing a program of study. I settled on a master of arts program in religion because it offered most of what I wanted, including the sociology and history of religion and a study of ethics.

The idea of writing a book about the ethics of health care had long been dormant in my mind but began to take definite shape when I initiated a course in medicine, religion, and human values at the George Washington University School of Medicine in 1965. Some of the features of this course and some of the research I did in this area are described in chapter 12.

This book uses a historical approach to develop the traditions and principles which I believe are fundamental in dealing with current ethical issues, and I have selected certain problem areas for discussion because I perceive them as important. Some of these areas and issues are not often treated in this context; for example, the worlds of organized medicine and medical education. Nevertheless, they should concern all health-care professionals and especially physicians.

The real heart of my effort is to describe and develop the concept of the physician as a professional person and to show the importance of the concepts of stewardship, *philia* or brotherly love, and situation ethics as they relate to the health-care professional who would wrestle with current ethical issues. This is not a textbook describing all approaches to medical ethics; that has been ably written by others. It is a work intended to describe an approach based on love, tradition, and professionalism. Since it is the approach I favor, it will necessarily reveal some of my biases.

However, please note that I am not saying this is the only approach, nor do I feel compelled to defend it against all the criticisms that have been made or could be made nor to compare it with other approaches. Space does not permit such luxuries. However, in the interests of *philia*, I must recognize that there are many ethicists who will not agree with what I say and they may be right. However, the approach I describe seems logical and workable to me and the principles have resisted the ravages of time.

Too few articles or books on medical ethics are written by physicians although that number has increased in recent years. As yet most authors in this field seem to come from the disciplines of religion or philosophy, and although such authors have made invaluable contributions to ethical thinking, they still suffer from a formidable limitation: although they often contribute to the thinking involved in a medical decision, they thus far have not had to make the final decision. Although they may have been consulted as to whether the resuscitator should be turned off or not, it is the physician who has had to ultimately do it or order it done, and only he or she has fully experienced the stress and anguish that this may entail.

Medicine needs all the help it can get from the other professions, and there has been a growing insistence that more of the professions and laity be involved in certain decision-making processes. It is my hope that this trend may continue and finally become standard, for the physician should not be required to bear all of this crushing responsibility. Such collaboration is a mark of interprofessional maturity.

Because physicians are uniquely involved in medical ethics their education should prepare them to deal with ethical questions, but still too few of them are thus equipped. They need more preparation at least in medical school and preferably starting in premedical training. Fortunately, newer graduates in medicine have more training in what has been called the "soft" sciences, which, I suppose, would include medical ethics, and there has been a definite increased interest in this area by a limited number of practicing physicians and medical educators. However, it is equally apparent that the majority of the medical profession are either neutral, unknowing, or even hostile to what they perceive to be medical ethics.

Some ethicists have complained that I seem unaware of *all* the arguments for some ethical issues or that I make simplistic observations at times. These criticisms are probably valid: I do not claim to be an ethicist and fail to see why ethics must be abstruse or complex. As a practicing physician, I encounter many ethical problems, and I need practical guidance. I was concerned enough about my lack of ethical knowledge to obtain formal training in this area, and apply it to the nuts and bolts of everyday practice. By the same reasoning, those who decry my lack of formal ethical knowledge but who continue to be mere speculative medical ethicists would do well to gain some practical experience in the medical world.

The process of getting this book published would make a story of its own and one which points up some of the problems I will be discussing in the text. I was encouraged to write the first draft by a religion press which demanded that they alone be allowed to consider the manuscript. After several months of silence they announced that they declined publication because they did not have adequate marketing facilities within the medical field. In the course of submitting the manuscript to various other presses I quickly discovered that few comprehended what I was writing about. Thus, the medical presses considered the work to be religious or philosophical and one editor commented that we must face the fact that "ethics simply generates negativism among many physicians." The religion presses, of course, thought it was medical. The university presses thought it was a "trade" book and the large trade publishers thought it was academic. The vanity presses didn't care about the audience.

It became increasingly obvious that some reviewers had read the manuscript very little or superficially because of their comments. One reviewer noted that I had "rambled off" into the area of medical education which was irrelevant to a book on medical ethics! By now, of course, I realized that I had done what, for some, was incomprehensible, if not unpardonable: I had crossed into several disciplines other than my own. I was now accustomed to being suspect by many physicians because of my training in religion and equally so by some religionists who regarded me as an intruder but I was almost totally unprepared by the lack of understanding shown by some reviewers and publishers. It is a tribute, I think, to Greenwood and their reviewers that they did see what I was trying to do and they came through with many valuable suggestions.

The "Hippocratic legacy" in the title is the catch-phrase I am using for the total body of ethical tradition in medicine, including contributions from religion such as stewardship and care for all those in need. Thus, Hippocrates may or may not be directly involved with this legacy, but his name has come to be synonymous with medical ethics so that such usage seems fitting.

I wish to acknowledge the help of many for their criticism and suggestions; some of which were hard to accept. Particular thanks are due Joseph Fletcher, John G. Fox, Mary McCaulley, Pat Robinson, Harry Yeide, Robert C. Derbyshire, and the unknown reviewer of the first draft. I also wish to thank the library staff of the Medical University of South Carolina and the Eastern Virginia Medical School.

MEDICAL STEWARDSHIP

CHAPTER 1

ANCIENT SOURCES

Health-care professionals have an obvious if often neglected role in current ethical issues. There are certain important traditions, roles, and concepts that should characterize the ethical physician or other health-care professional of our time. These concepts, including *philia* or neighborly love, stewardship, and professional traditions will be traced from the medieval guilds and universities to the present. I will examine the kind of person that society expects the physician to be and look at some of the codes, precepts, and oaths that have helped to shape this physician.

Love for one's neighbor is absolutely fundamental to the thesis of medical ethics I wish to develop. This type of love is known as C-love or *caritas* (from the Latin) from which comes our English word "charity," and *agape* or *philia* from the Greek. *Philia* is the word used by Dr. Entralgo to describe concerned friendship on the part of the physician for the patient and probably best connotes the type of love with which we are concerned.[1] *Philia* love is not sexual but is selfless and demands nothing in return; it is the type of love that should prevail between siblings or what we call brotherly love. *Philia* is used throughout this book and is often seen in English words of Greek ancestry such as philanthropy, or love for mankind.

What kind of person should a physician be? From the records of virtually all ancient cultures we find that the physician is expected to be a person of good will, good character, and good conduct; dedicated to his art or craft in which he possesses adequate skills and knowledge. Such expectations are reflected in an oath for the Hindu physician from ancient India and a Chinese code for physicians written in the seventh century A.D. but probably based on much older tradition.[2]

There was a proclivity in many ancient cultures for making gods out of outstanding physicians; thus, the Greeks ultimately deified Asklepios, a physician of Homeric times (1,200 B.C.), because of his legendary goodness and healing powers. The ancient Egyptians similarly deified Imhotep, a physician and architect of around 2,800 B.C. The ancient East Indian and Chinese cultures also had their physician-gods.[3] The reasons for this phenomenon are probably complex, but two factors seemed to prevail: (1) medicine and religion came from common roots as demonstrated by the medicine man-priest of primitive cultures and (2) the tendency to ascribe healing powers to divine sources. For example, from the Jews of the third century B.C., we have these observations:

Honor the doctor for his services, for the Lord created him. His skills come from the Most High, and he is rewarded by kings. The doctor's knowledge gives him high standing and wins him the admiration of the great. The Lord has created medicines from the earth, and a sensible man will not disparage them.[4]

Notice that in the above I have omitted any mention of *philia* or friendship on the part of the physician for his patient as a standard expectation of society. Many ancient sources seem content if the physician had love or *philia* for his art and maintained a certain decorum toward the patient. This is not to suggest that *philia* was lacking in ancient physicians but to suggest that the emphasis was different.

First hints of the importance of *philia* in the therapeutic relationship originated in the classical period of ancient Greece (fifth and fourth centuries B.C.).[5] From this era came the unique Hippocratic Oath which appears to have been taken by certain new physicians and stipulates certain norms of conduct. Although this oath has been traditionally ascribed to Hippocrates, the scholarly research by Ludwig Edelstein indicates that it most probably originated much later in the fourth century B.C. from an older cult of healers known as the Pythagoreans.[6] Regardless of the true source, the oath has some very important implications for medical ethics and stands as a monument of recorded concern by physicians for their patients.

The Hippocratic Oath is comprised of two sections; the first is concerned with the obligations of the person taking the oath to his teachers and colleagues, and the second part is concerned with the welfare of his patient. The text of the oath reproduced here is that used by Edelstein.

OATH

I swear by Apollo Physician and Asclepius and Hygieia and Panaceia and all the gods and goddesses, making them my witnesses, that I will fulfil according to my ability and judgment this oath and this covenant:

To hold him who has taught me this art as equal to my parents and to live my life in partnership with him, and if he is in need of money to give him a share of mine, and to regard his offspring as equal to my brothers in male lineage and to teach them this art—if they desire to learn it—without fee and covenant; to give a share of precepts and oral instruction and all the other learning to my sons and to the sons of him who has instructed me and to pupils who have signed the covenant and have taken an oath according to the medical law, but to no one else.

I will apply dietetic measures for the benefit of the sick according to my ability and judgment; I will keep them from harm and injustice.

I will neither give a deadly drug to anybody if asked for it, nor will I make a suggestion to this effect. Similarly I will not give to a woman an abortive remedy. In purity and holiness I will guard my life and my art.

I will not use the knife, not even on sufferers from stone, but will withdraw in favor of such men as are engaged in this work.

Whatever houses I may visit, I will come for the benefit of the sick, remaining free of all intentional injustice, of all mischief and in particular of sexual relations with both female and male persons, be they free or slaves.

What I may see or hear in the course of the treatment or even outside of the treatment in regard to the life of men, which on no account one must spread abroad, I will keep to myself holding such things shameful to be spoken about.

If I fulfil this oath and do not violate it, may it be granted to me to enjoy life and art, being honored with fame among all men for all time to come; if I transgress it and swear falsely, may the opposite of all this be my lot.

The first portion of the oath emphasizes the brotherhood of the physicians and respect for one's teachers as reflected in the several obligations and attitudes which one physician should hold for another.

The second portion deals with the doctor-patient relationship and is important for two reasons: first, the high calling of the profession demands high personal conduct of the physician, "in purity and holiness I will guard my life and my art;" secondly, because for the first time there are many concerns expressed for the patient's welfare. *Philia*, not mentioned by name, seems implied, and it is clear that the person taking the oath should feel that his calling is a very special one linked intimately with the care of a fellow human. Further, the advocacy role of the physician is expressed in the statement that the physician will keep his patient free from harm and injustice. This role of advocacy, common in the legal profession, is often forgotten in medicine. A reverence for life is expressed in the prohibition against giving an instrument for abortion, a practice that was widespread at the time. Further, information gathered in the course of patient care should not be revealed to others. The ethics of professional competence were implied in the admonition against using the knife, but rather leaving such work to those who were skilled at it.

Edelstein tells us that the oath was not widely accepted or practiced at the time of its formulation. One reason was that there were several competing cults of medicine, each with its own practices and beliefs, as well as that of the Pythagoreans, who alone banned abortion and suicide. Most physicians of the period were performing abortions and providing poisons for those who contemplated suicide. Edelstein makes the point that the medical ethics of this Golden Age of Greece consisted almost entirely of duty to or love of one's craft or were involved with medical etiquette and were concerned with what he calls the "outer performance" of physicians.

However, in the later Hellenic period the sentiments of the oath encountered growing support from Greek humanism and philosophy, especially Stoicism, and were ultimately reinforced and enriched by important concepts from Judaism and Christianity. This led to what Edelstein calls the second stage of Greek medical ethics, which was concerned with the inner attitude and intent of the physician. The final product was a blend of outer performance and inner intent, which was gradually adopted by a growing number of Greco-Roman physicians.

Although the oath was unique in its time for its emphasis on concern, if not *philia*, for the individual patient, it registered no concern for society in general. Its preoccupation with the duty owed the patient may have been a factor in the hallowing of the traditional one to one doctor-patient relationship and the consequent neglect of medico-social concerns for the group. By distinction, ancient Chinese medicine was concerned with the care of society as well as the individual.[7]

Despite its limitations, the Hippocratic Oath stands as a monument of recorded concern for the patient and the obligations of the physician. The emphasis of the oath on the four Cs of character, competence, caring, and confidentiality have been recognized throughout the ages as enduring qualities for the ethical physician. As Edelstein reminds us:

As time went on, the Hippocratic Oath became the nucleus of all medical ethics. In all countries, in all epochs in which monotheism in its purely religious or its more secularized form, was the adopted creed, the Hippocratic Oath was applauded as the embodiment of truth. Not only Jews and Christians, but the Arabs, the medieval doctors, men of the Renaissance, scientists of the Enlightenment, and scholars of the 19th century embraced the ideals of the Oath.[8]

A modern version of the oath is the Declaration of Geneva (1948), which is reproduced in the appendix.

Besides the oath there is an abundance of other medical writings traditionally ascribed to Hippocrates that is known collectively as the *Hippocratic Corpus*. This collection includes such titles as *Epidemics, Law, Aphorisms, Precepts, Decorum,* and *On the Physician* and most probably represents writings by Hippocrates as well as others from the time of Hippocrates down to the Christian era. Exact proof of authorship is lacking, but the dating is reasonably accurate and the writings themselves reflect the best of Greek scientific medicine as well as the humanism that derived from the major philosophical schools of the period.

An important statement comes from the *Precepts*, Sec. VI, which is often quoted in fragmentary form. The passage in question reads: "Sometimes give your services for nothing.... And if there be any opportunity of serving one who is a stranger in financial straits, give full assistance to all such. For where there is love of man, there is also love of the art." The service tradition of medicine is thus a very old one, indeed, and the same advice is found in ancient medical writings from China and India. There were writers from the same era who were equally convinced that "where there is no fee there is no skill," but the service tradition has endured through the centuries to our time. Despite some controversy about the contextual relationship of the phrase "love of the art," there is no escaping an intimate relationship between love as *philia* and the practice of medicine, and therefore, the physician sometimes provides care without charge.

Another familiar expression that has puzzled me for some years, the so-called first rule of medicine, is "first, do not harm." Often seen in its Latin form as *primum non nocere*, it undoubtedly is a Roman corruption of another saying attributed to Hippocrates and is found in his *Epidemics* Sec. II, where it reads: "As to disease, make a habit of two things: to help or at least do no harm." This is certainly more reasonable and in keeping with the *philia* suggested by the oath and as stated in the above quotation from the *Precepts*.

Hippocrates has traditionally been associated with the healing cult of Asklepios whose members were known as Asklepiads. However, according to Major, there are some problems with this traditional view.[9] Hippocrates was born and practiced his art on the island of Kos, which was the site of a major Asklepion or healing center. However, the Koan Asklepion appears to have been built several centuries after Hippocrates's birth, and further, he was the first Greek physician to separate medicine from religion, which played an important part in the healing rituals of the Asklepiads. This separation was a necessary and pivotal point in the development of scientific medicine, but it also helped to create another problem which is ironical: medicine and religion sprang from a common root and shared some important truths which would be obscured for centuries. There would be recurrent enmity between medical science and religion, which is even now not totally resolved.

Notwithstanding Hippocrates's views on the separation of religion from medicine, he felt strongly about the role of philosophy in medicine and stated that the physician-philosopher was the equivalent of the gods.[10] It seems clear from this and his other writings that he felt the physician must be a well-rounded person and not a mere technician; a sentiment that has been echoed in our times.

There is no question of the great influence of the Hippocratic writings on the development of medical ethics, and even without proven authorship of these writings, Hippocrates is important for being the founder and the greatest practitioner of the Koan school of scientific medicine.

Now we'll consider some of the important Judaic and Christian contributions to ethical thought.

For the Jews there was but one source of healing; God, who had created both the skills of the physician and medicines from the earth. Sickness or other afflictions were not God's punishment for sins but might be permitted for some purpose man could not fathom. Mankind was to obey the two Great Commandments; to love God and to love one's neighbor as oneself. However, the prophets made it clear that God's people did not always heed these commandments.

It is sometimes forgotten that Christianity began as an internal reform movement within Judaism. Jesus, as a believing Jew, emphasized that the faith was summarized in the two Great Commandments, and he went an important step further by equating their meaning; man shows his love of God by loving his neighbor.[11] Also, in the Gospel according to John, the faithful are exhorted to love one another as God loves them. Naturally enough, the Hippocratic Oath found ready acceptance among early Christians because of its expressions of concern, if not *philia*, for a fellow human.

Christians thus had a duty or charge to love one another that found quick expression in the care of widows, orphans, the poor, and the sick. Hospices for those in need were established everywhere and ultimately led to the establishment of the medieval hospitals with which the Church has been continuously associated. Whereas most Greek physicians would not treat patients deemed incurable or incapable of being fit citizens, Christians cared for lepers, cripples, and others who would have ordinarily been left to die. In their *agape* love context, early Christians could use Greek medicine as the best of its time and equate the Hippocratic Oath with their own love ethic. The question of whether it is truly ethical to prolong life in certain cases did not seem to trouble the early Christians perhaps because they were reacting against the perceived callousness of the time. In their *agape* fervor, some Christians even venerated Galen (ca. 200 A.D.), the last great physician of the Hippocratic or Koan school because of his great skill and knowledge.[12] Interestingly, the old healing cult of Asklepios with which Hippocrates is often associated continued to flourish and compete with Christianity for many years.

In addition, there were many references in the Church and Scripture to Christ as the Great Physician and many healing miracles narrated in the New Testament so there was a natural alliance between Christianity and medicine as epitomizing love as *philia* or *agape*. Tragically, the later Church would periodically denounce Greek scientific medicine as "pagan," a view that created a chronic enmity between medicine and religion. Thus, the emperor Theodosius destroyed the old Greek healing centers, or Asklepions, and the emperor Justinian closed the two great universities and medical schools of his time, all in the name of Christian piety. The Jewish scriptural wisdom that there was but one author of knowledge and healing would be lost by the Church for many centuries.

Stewardship is an important concept for physicians. In another example of cross-cultural borrowing and blending, the early Christian Church borrowed the Greek notion of stewardship and expanded it to a central position in their agapism. The Greek work *oikonomos* in the New Testament means "overseer" or "steward" and from it comes our modern word "economy." The overseer or steward is one who is expected to prudently manage or administer the property or goods of another. This implies, as in the New Testament parable of the talents, that a steward must strive to improve that over which he has care. In this parable, a sum of money or talents was left with each of three stewards by the lord of the manor. In his absence, two of the stewards wisely invested the money and increased the total. The third steward buried his for safety and did nothing further. When the lord returned and asked for an accounting, he commended the first two and rebuked the third.

This theme was developed by the Church so that stewardship ultimately postulated that every person, as a steward, receives a lifetime allocation of gifts from the Creator. Among these gifts are life, love, fellowship, intelligence, and the resources of this natural world. We hold these gifts in trust for our lifetime and are expected to make a final accounting of how we used them. The expectation, in this context, is that we shall have used them wisely and worked for their improvement; that is, the quality of life itself must not only be preserved but improved.

The stewardship doctrine further states that everyone must work within the confines of what has been called the "divine economy," which is the masterplan for this planet and the cosmos as revealed by God. Man must therefore constantly work toward a more complete understanding of that divine economy and strive for a harmonious relationship within it. It was commonly held by the Greek intellectuals of the classical period that the *physis* or nature of man must be in harmony with *physis* or nature in general; disease was a manifestation of disharmony. Christian stewardship thus embraced a world view that had long been held in the Greco-Roman world. To truly love one's neighbor one must exercise good stewardship in order that the neighbor not be harmed and that his life might be made better. "Neighbor" in this context includes all citizens of this planet.

There are important implications of stewardship for the physician. It is obvious that physicians have been given more than an average share of "talents," and therefore more is expected from them. The medical profession is inherently involved with improving the quality of life in the care of patients but must also see to the provision of adequate health care for everyone. Stewardship is a key function of the physician; it requires one to act in the best interests of the patient, regardless of one's personal bias. This is the ancient responsibility one assumes on becoming a member of the medical profession.

What kind of an ethic or ethics should flow from this stewardship role? The preface states that ethics involves reflection and decision as to how we act or refrain from acting towards others. Throughout the ages men have wrestled with the problem of how to approach ethical conduct, and many different methods have been devised. For example, in some ethical schemes the motive or intention behind an act is all-important, while for others, the consequence of an action is the ultimate concern. Others believe that both of these views are important. There are also ethics that are based on religion, on nature, on a legal system or a completely lawless, anything-goes approach; others operate on pleasure as a guiding principle; still others, out of duty. There are systems based on malice and others based on love, some favor the individual while others are interested in the good of the group. The systems and their various combinations are almost limitless.

Joseph Fletcher has done much in his writing and lecturing to popularize what is known as "situation ethics," an ethical approach based on *agape* or *philia* love, with each ethical situation being considered on its own merits and circumstances and the greatest concern being shown for the consequences. This approach does not ignore suitable norms of ethical conduct that have been tested by time nor the collected wisdom of the ages. However, such norms and wisdom are never absolutely binding but serve only as guidelines. For the situationist, love is the only absolute, and within its context there is neither inflexible rule nor anarchy but rather a pervasive *philia* which takes into account all of the factors in a given ethical situation.

In Fletcher's view, the situationist is not so much concerned with what is "right" or "good" but what is *fitting* in any given case.[13] This orientation is easily carried over into medical ethics where that which helps or improves the patient is fitting and therefore the desirable course of action. On the subject of euthanasia, for example, a given legalistic approach might say that the termination of a human life, however defined and for whatever reason, is always wrong, while a lawless or antinomian system might say that such an action is neither right nor wrong, and a decision should be left entirely to the individual or group concerned. Situation ethics might hold that there must be an abiding reverence for human life, and therefore terminating a life may be wrong in some circumstances, permissible in others, or be an act of love in still others. There is a long tradition that the circumstances surrounding a given action may modify the judgment of that action.

The situation approach is not without fault either, for the best-intentioned situationist can err lovingly and thus cause harm. Critics have also raised the question of who is to decide what the situationist should love? I think that this is missing the point, however, for it is not a question of whom or what should be loved but rather that *philia* or *agape* should always be exercised. And when love is supreme, as Fletcher warns us it must be, then the situationist will welcome criticism, reflect on his decisions and mistakes, and continue to work for optimal consequences for each ethical problem. Yes, mistakes will be made in such an approach, but where there is a loving concern for others there will be a powerful force for correction and improvement. It is situation ethics which, in my opinion, best suits the stewardship role and results in applied *philia* in the daily practice of medicine.

With the death of Galen in the early third century A.D., Greek scientific medicine gradually declined in the West and passed into the Dark Ages after the collapse of Rome. The bulk of the Hippocratic and some of the Galenic writings survived in the East and were well-known to the Byzantine, Persian, and Islamic empires but unfortunately, these would not be recovered by the West until the high Middle Ages. It was equally unfortunate that the fragmentary writings of Galen, which did survive in the West, would be venerated and remain unchallenged as the standard of medical practice in the West until the classical writings of the Hippocratic school were brought back in the twelfth century A.D.

In the interim of several centuries, the best medicine was taught and practiced in the East, in both the Byzantine and Islamic empires. The caliphs of the Islamic world (700-1100 A.D.)

were zealous collectors of all written knowledge of the time, including writings from Greece, India, China, and Egypt. In this stimulating period, intellectual activity flourished among physicians and scholars of all Eastern religions and cultures. Two physicians who lived and wrote within the influence of the Western Caliphate of Islam are worth noting.

Isaac Israel, a Jewish physician of the ninth century A.D., has left us his *Fifty Admonitions to the Physician*, which are instructive for the type of conduct desirable for a physician. By the nature of his work and study, the physician is set aside from other men. He must be neither boastful nor hasty in judgment or action except in acute need. He should not promise a cure, for only death is a certainty. It is as important for a physician to preserve health as it is to treat disease. Throughout Israel's work one sees the influence of the writings attributed to Hippocrates and several references to Galen as the Lord of Physicians.[14]

Al-Ruhawi, an Arabic physician of the same period, stated that a physician should be a man of good moral character, generous, dignified, and not given to pettiness. He should strive to be clean on the inside as well as the outside. Although al-Ruhawi wrote as an Arab, his biographer, Levey, tells us he was probably a Christian.[15] In regard to competence, al-Ruhawi felt there was merit in the custom of the ancient Greek physicians to review the conduct of a physician whose patient had died. If they found the physician negligent in the care of the patient, he was put to death.[16] Peer review, as this procedure is called, was not common in antiquity so far as we know, although there are many comments on the physician's need to be competent. It is quite possible that al-Ruhawi had a corrupt translation or copy of Plato's *Laws* wherein it is stated that physicians found guilty of deliberately causing death or harm to a patient would be put to death. Amundsen tells us that there is no evidence for legal liability of the physician for malpractice in classical Greece, but there were other powerful deterrents: (1) the enormous importance of maintaining one's good reputation, (2) love of one's art or *philotekne*, which made it imperative to help rather than harm the patient and, (3) the prevailing custom of refusing to accept hopeless cases and hence avoiding blame for death or disability.[17] However, many authors of this classical period agreed that a physician charged with improper conduct qua physician should be tried only by other physicians or lay persons educated in medicine.

There is strong evidence from antiquity that self-regulation of physicians, oaths, codes of conduct, and peer review, were not always adequate to insure there would be ethical and competent practitioners of the art. From ancient Babylon of 2,000 B.C. we have the Code of Hammurabi, the earliest known set of laws dealing with the conduct and fees charged by surgeons. Specific penalties were imposed for infraction of these laws, which appear to have been written because of perceived misconduct among the practitioners of the time. This question of ethical and competent practitioners appears to have been and remains a problem for all cultures, including ours. Although we have no record of medical ethics, codes, oaths, or self-regulation, from this period in Babylon, it is reasonable to suppose that such voluntary restraints did exist, for they did in virtually all early civilizations. Assuming that some ethical controls did exist in early Babylon as elsewhere, it is obvious they did not uniformly succeed, since regulation was imposed by the state. Since 2,000 B.C. there have been recurrent episodes of concern by states in various times and places for the regulation of medicine, and the result has been the passage of various laws.[18] It is evident that the health-care profession has not always, if ever, been equal to the task of self-regulation. Can true *philia* ethics succeed where laws and oaths have not?

In order to determine how physicians should act toward one another and toward the persons for whom they care I have scanned several centuries of ancient cultures. It is clear that from earliest times and in various cultures there is amazing agreement that the physician was expected to be someone very special, of good character and manners, charitable, competent and knowledgable in the art of medicine and dedicated to that art. As time passed on there was a gradually increasing emphasis on the need for the physician to exercise *philia* for the patient and a universal service tradition usually manifested by free care to those in need.

CHAPTER 2

THE MEANING OF THE PROFESSIONAL PERSON

What constitutes being a professional and what are the characteristics of the professional person? The term "professional" has various definitions which has caused a blurring of what constitutes a professional person. For example, one hears about a professional burglar or that prostitution is the oldest profession.[1] In sports, the earning of money for playing a particular sport is what distinguishes a "pro" from an amateur.

Scribonius Largus, a physician-author of the first century A.D. may have been the first to use the term "profession" in reference to medicine and with particular reference to the ethical role of the physician. Edelstein tells us that Scribonius had a clear realization of the medical humanism inherent in the task of physicians; this humanism and sympathy on the part of the physician is due everyone equally.[2] Furthermore, this humanism is not just friendliness toward the patient, but rather proficiency and benevolence toward all men. Scribonius uses the Latin *humanitas*, which Edelstein likens to "love of mankind" or the Greek *philanthropos*. Love of humanity and sympathy are special obligations of the physician, and they are required of him by medicine itself, just as competence and knowledge are required. The physician must, then, possess skills and knowledge and exercise his moral responsibility or be derelict in his duty. Edelstein makes the important point that it is hardly by chance "Scribonius calls medicine not merely an art or a science but a *profession*." (italics mine)

This ancient use of the word "profession" to characterize medicine emphasized the ethical connotations of the art and closely approximated the Christian concept of "vocation" or "calling." This usage is similar to the phrase "to profess a faith" or to profess or acknowledge before the world a particular vocation or calling.

The development of the so-called "learned professions" had their beginnings in the emerging European universities of the twelfth century and consisted of law, medicine, and theology. The intimate relationship between these professions as a religious calling is underscored by the requirement that medical and law students had to take at least minor religious orders in the Church. From this time on, the professional person has been associated with a superior level of education and knowledge.

Paralleling the rise of the universities was the emergence of the medieval craft guilds. These voluntary associations of craftsmen in a given field were formed by motives of mutual interest, a desire to limit competition and to establish and maintain standards of training and performance. Hence, the guilds were characterized by being organized by standards of training and competence and machinery for maintaining that competence, that is, discipline. These attributes gradually merged with the concept of the learned professions and have come to be associated with the notion of a contemporary profession. However, there are other features as well.

In a thorough analysis of contemporary professions, Moore has described the following characteristics:

1. A total commitment to a calling, usually demanding full-time participation.
2. Organization
3. A high level of education
4. Clients
5. Individual autonomy and responsibility
6. A service orientation[3]

A true professional keeps his identity 24 hours a day; a profession is not a part-time occupation. Professions are organized; the physicians have their medical associations and the lawyers have their bar associations. A high level of education is necessary to provide knowledge not readily available or capable of being understood by all. Professions normally interact with clients for whom they provide services rather than goods.

A professional person has a high level of education and expertise in a field that is not easily available to a lay person. As a consequence, society has customarily awarded special recognition to professionals by allowing them wide latitude or autonomy in their provision of services to clients. In granting such autonomy, society has indicated that it also expects a commensurate degree of responsibility for self-regulation from the professional. A professional may thus be viewed as one in whom a certain amount of public trust has been vested, a trust that says he will act in the best interests of his client.

However, not all professionals have kept that public trust. In an effort to minimize the individual abuse of trust, a group of professional colleagues may provide peer review of the actions of the individual; a procedure that can be effective self-regulation. The autonomy-responsibility of the individual professional may then pass in some degree to the professional group, although it is also possible for the group to abuse its privilege of autonomy.

The service orientation that is characteristic of a profession means that a part of its efforts is directed toward public good without renumeration. This is a strong tradition in medicine going back to pre-Christian times. This factor is also taken into account by society in the conferring of a privileged status on the professional. Often neglected or obscured, this ancient tradition places service to others as a primary goal of the craft with monetary gain as secondary. This does not mean that material gain is wrong but that it should come as a result of being fully professional, which includes placing an emphasis on service. The 1957 version of the Principles of Medical Ethics of the American Medical Association was virtually unchanged for 23 years. The first principle of the 1957 version stated:

The principal objective of the medical profession is to render service to humanity with full respect for the dignity of man. Physicians should merit the confidence of patients entrusted to their care, rendering to each a full measure of service and devotion.[4]

However, the Principles were revised by the AMA in 1980 and the first principle now reads: "A physician shall be dedicated to providing competent medical service with compassion and respect for human dignity."[5] I leave it to the reader to judge whether the service-first emphasis of the older version has not been deleted in this new one. It is clear to me that this emphasis has been dropped, and this represents danger to the future of the craft since it weakens a primary characteristic of the professional person. If the physician is to be fully professional, this traditional principle must continue to be honored. The current sentiment in this nation for medical care as a right for all rather than a privilege for some is in full accord with the service tradition of medicine. Both the 1957 and the 1980 versions of the Principles are contained in the appendices.

Another hallmark of the professions, especially law and medicine, is the role of advocacy. We are all accustomed to seeing lawyers in movies act as advocate for their clients. Although medicine is not usually considered in this light, the physician has an equally important role of being an advocate for the patient. The rights and opinions of the patient must be protected and respected, but there have been untold instances of physicians who have usurped these rights and opinions on the questionable grounds of knowing what was best for their patients.

The triad of organization, standards, and discipline of the professions grew out of the guild tradition of medieval Europe. The American Bar Association and the American Medical Association typify this organization. A primary purpose of professional organization is to set standards for training, competence, and conduct of members. Thus, at the first real meeting of the AMA in 1847, the principal items of business were the establishment of a code of ethics and the establishment of requirements for medical education and training. Disciplinary measures to ensure conformity to the standards of competence and conduct are also important functions of the organization. When the three professional characteristics of responsibility, competence, and discipline are blended with the ancient tradition of service-in-love, we then have the elements of the physician as a professional. To be a professional in the true sense implies that the physician must constantly observe this full tradition. Furthermore, if one's professional organization gets preoccupied with the politics of preserving its own vested interests, then one may fairly question whether such an organization is truly professional.

Following the medieval period came the Renaissance and the Age of Enlightenment with pragmatic philosophers and social reformers calling attention to the many who were abused and disadvantaged by the conditions accompanying emerging industrial societies.[6] Certain economic philosophies showed that man alone was responsible for how the goods of the world were distributed and that *unchecked* capitalism would lead to its own collapse. Such discoveries and thinking gradually led to social and governmental reforms which have continued to the present, including our current social medicine programs.[7]

Out of the Age of Enlightenment also came the first treatise on medical ethics of the modern era. Thomas Percival, a general medical practitioner of Manchester, England, was requested by the Manchester Infirmary to write a set of rules governing the conduct of its medical staff. Published in 1803, Percival's *Medical Ethics* was more a compendium of rules than a system of ethics, but it went far beyond its commission as a book of rules and supplied some sorely needed ethical principles and a workable code of conduct for physicians. As Burns ably puts it:

The hospital was a new stage for the expression of ethical conflicts by British physicians, surgeons, and apothecaries. The oaths of antiquity, the moral maxims of the traditional guilds, and the legally binding statutory responses to these professional hierarchies were no longer satisfactory.[8]

All things considered, Percival's book met this need surprisingly well.

Percival was concerned with the conduct of a physician in four areas: (1) as a gentleman, (2) in interactions between physicians, (3) in the doctor-patient relationship and (4) in interaction with the public.

The personal values and conduct of the physician, Percival felt, should be those of the classical tradition. In the matter of interaction with other physicians, the welfare of the patient should be paramount. Hence, a physician should question the competence of another only through formal channels except in an emergency where interference would be a duty. The physician had an obligation to the public to obey the laws and to perform certain public medical duties honestly and faithfully in return for certain privileges and status conferred on him by the state. This is in accord with the special status given the physician as a professional.

In the matter of interaction with the patient, the physician should respect his opinions and feelings. Fake or secret remedies were not to be used. The physician should consider the patient's personal problems as well as the medical ones. It is quite clear from Burns's article that the welfare of the patient was Percival's first consideration. Although Percival admitted several defects in his book, it was obviously written in full accord with what has been discussed here as true professionalism. This work is epochal because it formed the basis of American and British medical ethics for many decades.

CHAPTER 3

FORGING AN ETHICAL DEVICE

One cannot escape the consensus of many cultures, spanning millennia, that a physician should be a superior person in competence, character, and conduct. From classical Greece came the Hippocratic Corpus, including the oath, which united science and humanism in medicine. Over the years Greek humanism became increasingly blended with the Judeo-Christian imperative of neighborly love and the concept of stewardship. This doctrine of stewardship emphasized advocacy, service, and wise use of the Creator's gifts and recognized that the physician, as steward, was but an agent of one ultimate source of healing. The physician was a natural personage for the stewardship role enacted in the spirit of *philia* for all those in need of medical care; an attitude consistent with the continuing tradition of the Church to care for all those in need.

From the medieval period came the beginnings of the modern learned professions, including medicine, and from the guilds came the emphasis on organization, standards, and discipline. These contributions from the guilds were important since they recognized man's weakness as an individual and sought to overcome it by forming associations with common interests and ways to protect the group standards and maintain the quality of their goods and services. Such internal regulaton was really early peer review and set the guilds apart from the general public since, theoretically, outside regulation by the state was not needed so long as self-regulation was effective. To some degree, the guilds put into their governance some of the precepts of the Hippocratic Oath: brotherhood, competence, and implied danger for those who transgressed the norms and rules of the organization.

The publication of Percival's *Medical Ethics* in 1803 was remark-able because it drew together for the first time most of the ancient traditons of medical ethics and the characteristics of the professional person of our modern period. The codified approach used by Percival persisted in this country until 1957, at which time it was supplanted by ethical principles. Still, many health care professionals continue to view medical ethics as a collection of do's and don'ts.

In order to create a useful mental picture, I propose the follow-ing model: one may conceive of a wheel which represents the world. The hub of the wheel is represented by *philia* love. From that hub radiates the four spokes or rays of responsibility, com-petence, discipline, and service reaching out to the entire world and always rooted in the central *philia*. Without *philia* as the pervasive driving force, the symbol is without meaning, just as a wheel is useless without a hub. Accordingly, in any encounter with an ethical problem in medicine, we must seek solutions in understanding and *philia*.

CHAPTER 4

THE ETHICS OF MEDICAL ORGANIZATIONS

Although a number of medical organizations exist in this country, when one thinks of "medical organization" the American Medical Association usually comes to mind; a name virtually synonymous with organized medicine. There is also the much smaller National Medical Association originally founded by black physicians because until recently they were barred from membership in some state societies of the AMA. Organizations like the AMA and NMA constitute a type known as medical societies and are composed of physicians voluntarily joined together for broad mutual interests.

There are other medical organizations to be sure; for example, the medical specialty boards which certify that qualified physicians have minimum standards of competence and knowledge within a given specialty. And there are the Association of American Medical Colleges and various academies and colleges. The so-called academies and colleges function much like the medical societies but on a reduced scale, and their membership is normally made up of those who follow a certain medical specialty. Each of these medical organizations obviously has special interests and concerns as well as certain common ones. However, it is the AMA with which we are most concerned here, for it is the

AMA which has been called "the voice of American medicine," and certainly it is the largest and most powerful medical organization in this country. Therefore I have selected the AMA as a "case study," although many of my remarks apply to other medical organizations as well.

The AMA is big business: In 1976 it had an annual budget of 42.9 million dollars and has admitted, at various times, to being the biggest lobby in the nation's capital. It is also representative of many American physicians and thus has ethical obligations in both of these areas.

Historically, the first concerns of the AMA were the ethical conduct of physicians and standards for medical education. Since its inception in 1847, the AMA has maintained interest in both of these areas, but medical education has received the bulk of its attention. But let us now look at some of the stated objectives of the AMA. From the AMA's *Model Constitution and By-laws for a Medical Society* under Article II we read:

PURPOSES

The purpose of this Society shall be to form an organization of the physicians of _____ County, so that by frequent meetings and full and frank interchange of views they may secure such intelligent unity in every phase of their labor as will elevate and make effective the opinions of the profession in all scientific, public policy and health, material and social affairs, *to the end that the profession may receive that respect and support within its own ranks and from the community to which its honorable history and great achievement entitle it.* (italics mine)

I confess to having a great deal of difficulty with this section. It seems to be self-seeking and delusory. I cannot believe that a primary purpose of organized medicine is to achieve "that respect and support" to which it feels it is entitled. True, there has been occasional greatness of some individuals in the history of medicine but a collective greatness? No. Tributes such as respect and support should be a secondary consequence of following the primary goals of medicine as described in our ethical traditions; namely, the performance of competent and responsible service to all in need, given in a spirit of *philia*. Tributes, like material gain, should be secondary rewards of medicine resulting from the faithful performance of the primary objective.

Moving on to chapter 2 of the same *Model Constitution and By-laws* we read the following:

POWERS AND DUTIES

Section 1. Purpose—This Society shall encourage among the members of the profession the interchange of views on all phases of professional advancement to equip such members of the profession to serve society and promote public health, maintain a program of scientific education for members of the Society, advance the standard of medical practice and insure observance of the ideals *and* the ethics of the medical profession.

Dropping down to section 4, we read:

Community Responsibilities—This Society shall endeavor to educate its members to the belief that a physician should be a leader in his community, in character, in learning, in dignified and manly bearing, and in courteous and open treatment of his brother physicians, to the end that the profession may occupy that place in its own and the public estimation to which it is entitled.

From the foregoing quotation it is clear that the AMA ideologically encourages its members to "serve society and promote public health," to maintain an educational program, to advance the standards of medical practice, and "insure" observance of the ideals of the medical profession. I have some uneasiness about this because it is unclear to me just how one may "insure observance of ideals," but the general intent of the clause appears to be an approach to the ideal of ethical conduct, however that may be defined. There is less ambiguity in the stipulation that members are expected to provide "courteous and open treatment" of brother physicians.

Some additional goals are delineated in a later brochure published by the AMA entitled *Make the Most of your A. M. A.* A few of these are of special interest: " ... To attract increasing numbers of capable people into medicine and the other healthcare professions." To foster programs "that will encourage medical and health personnel to serve voluntarily in the areas of need for medical care." To develop methods "that will moderate the costs of good medical and health care." To maintain "the highest level of ethics and professional standards among all members of the medical profession." To continue "to provide leadership and guidance to the medical profession of the world in meeting the health needs of changing populations."

In a 1965 AMA brochure the following statement appears: "The medical profession is dedicated to the provision of medical service for all, regardless of ability to pay. On the average, a physician donates about 12½ percent of his time to providing free care." So much for the goals; what about the fulfillment?

The medical profession has a long tradition of concern for medical education dating back at least to the Hippocratic Oath, and this is entirely consistent with the ethical traditions or spokes of responsibility and competence on my symbolic wheel of the world. Although the AMA has had an abiding interest in medical education from its first days, the reasons for this interest were not always altruistic. The role of the AMA as a real power in this area began in 1904 with the creation of its Council on Medical Education. Because of the lack of standardization in medical education and the questionable quality of many medical schools, the council commissioned the Carnegie Foundation for the Advancement of Teaching to do a comprehensive survey of the medical schools in this country. The result was the epochal "Flexner Report," named after the educator who did the actual survey.[1] No one at the time could envision the impact of this report, which is still felt seventy years later. The most immediate and dramatic effect of Abraham Flexner's report was to aid the Council on Medical Education in its efforts to close the unsatisfactory medical schools; the total number of schools in the United States dropped from 160 in 1900 to 76 in 1930. Only those schools with an "A" or acceptable rating remained in business after 1939.

There is no question that the medical schools of this country needed periodic evaluation with a weeding out or upgrading of the bad ones. The AMA arrogated this task to itself early in this century. Undoubtedly many physicians involved with this work were concerned only with the improvement of medical education and the quality of medical care; a traditional and laudable motivation. But there is also considerable evidence that the AMA embarked on a course of professional contraception to reduce the number of new physicians in this country for purely economic reasons.[2] Not only was the total number of medical schools reduced, but beginning in the thirties, the AMA was beginning to coerce the remaining schools to accept fewer students. Since the Council on Medical Education was still solely responsible for the rating of the schools, it was able to get its message across. The resulting shortage of physicians reached crisis proportions in the 1950s, necessitating a crash program for new schools, which the AMA only grudgingly supported.[3]

Although the inferior schools were forced out of business by the Flexner Report, there was little or no encouragement or funds to replace them with good ones. Five of the nation's seven black schools ultimately shut down, partly as a result of the report and partly from lack of funds. A disproportionate number of schools also closed which had been open to working-class youths, many of whom had attended as part-time students; a fact noted by Flexner himself. A possibly unforeseen result was to keep the bulk of new physicians white and upper-middle class; a condition which still largely prevails.[4] For a long time the AMA opposed federal aid to medical schools, thus depriving many poor students with good qualifications of a chance to enter medicine. Although the AMA has endeavored for years to provide scholarship and loan funds through private gifts, they have not been adequate, and it has finally conceded that support for medical education is required from federal, state, and private sources.

One remarkable fact is that no one seems to have questioned (until recently) the solo role of the AMA in accrediting our medical schools which it held until 1942. Only then did it share this function with the Association of American Medical Colleges in what is known as the Liason Committee on Medical Education. (LCME). Medical education in this country had been such a swamp that there was general rejoicing when the AMA appointed itself to the role of reform agent. This rejoicing would blind most to the dangers inherent in the unchecked manipulations of the AMA in medical education, which would create a physician shortage and make a medical education difficult for the disadvantaged student. Only recently was this role challenged by the Federal Trade Commission as a conflict of interest with the recommendation to the United States Office of Education that the LCME's authority not be continued. As of now (1981) the AMA is still participating in this committee despite the FTC's recommendation. It is unclear why such a visible ethical and legal breach escaped public awareness and correction for as long as it has. The role the AMA has played is a splendid example of the exercise of a commendable ethical tradition on the part of organized medicine, that of maintaining educational standards, with an equally splendid example of abuse of that function for selfish reasons.

After the AMA reorganized itself into a powerful federation early in this century, it was fortunate to count a good number of social liberals and progressives in its hierarchy. During these early years, it worked long and hard for the passage of various health laws and protection of the public against quackery and drugs or foods of doubtful quality or safety. The AMA of those years did not hesitate to attack political machines, drug houses, or big business in general regarding questions of public health. The AMA supported the establishment of a comprehensive national health insurance program (NHI) such as had become popular in Europe in this period.[5] However, this all too brief golden age of the AMA collapsed at its annual 1920 meeting when a proposal for national health insurance was defeated by a determined and tightly knit minority that managed to permanently sabotage the proposal by some adroit manipulations. The mold was now hardened for the AMA to be the defender of the entrepreneurial fee for service system and adversary of socialized medicine, including any national health insurance scheme controlled by government, and that policy has prevailed to the present.

With the end of organized medicine's brief golden age began what has been called the Fishbein Era, named for Morris Fishbein, a physician who was the "spiritual" leader and the embodiment of the AMA for some 29 years. He had joined the AMA staff in 1912 as assistant editor of the *Journal of the A. M. A.* and rose to prominence at the 1920 meeting, where he worked with the forces which wanted the AMA to represent the fee-for-service crowd. A hero or a devil, depending on which camp you came from, Fishbein has been credited with holding medicine back in the nineteenth century for some forty years of the twentieth. The Fishbein success story was simple; it consisted in giving the members what they thought they wanted. The majority of physicians were in private practice charging fees for service, now the AMA had made it clear it opposed any national health insurance scheme which would alter the renumeration basis. What else was there to fear? This honeymoon relationship of the hierarchy to the membership was to continue for as long as Fishbein was at the helm. With the sharp and continuing reduction in the absolute numbers of practicing physicians and a parallel increase in the general population, the AMA membership in private practice soon realized they were in on a very good thing, namely, rising incomes. It is hard to quarrel with success. If the membership did not know what it wanted in other areas, Doctor Fishbein managed to tell them so well that his long reign was virtually unchallenged.[6] As editor of the *Journal* and later as senior statesman, he wielded enormous power and influence. Ironically, when the AMA was crusading against socialized medicine in 1949, Fishbein was ousted by the board of trustees because he was a "symbol of old, reactionary leadership."

The AMA is active in many aspects of medical education and participates, for example, in the accreditation of graduate medical education through membership on the Liason Committee for Graduate Medical Education. It also had been participating in the Liason Committee on Continuing Medical Education (LCCME), which accredits programs in this field for practicing physicians throughout the country. However, after a dispute with the other participants of the committee in 1979, the AMA withdrew its membership and announced it would do its own accrediting in this area. Planners of new programs have been forced to seek accreditation from both the AMA and the LCCME, since it is unclear which body they should choose. This is regretable, because there is a real need for a national coordinating body which can both reflect the educational needs and accredit and regulate the content of the swelling tide of programs in this field. Many of these programs appear to be of doubtful quality and are purely commercial. There is no question that the AMA likes to be in control of whatever committee on which it sits. What has happened to medicine's traditional spirit of fraternity and *philia*?

The AMA also has representation on the Coordinating Council on Medical Education (CCME) and participates in the annual Congress on Medical Education. The CCME is a long-needed collaborative effort of the American Board of Medical Specialties, the American Hospital Association, the AMA, and the Council on Medical Specialty Societies. In its relatively short history it has done much good work with study projects completed and going on in several fields including physician distribution, the role of foreign medical graduates, and the role of the primary care physician. A comparison of the good work the AMA is doing here with the power-hungry AMA in the preceding paragraph leaves no doubt as to which role is in accord with the *philia* spirit.

It seems fair to conclude that the AMA has been a Jekyll and Hyde in its interactions with medical education. Beginning with Fishbein, the AMA has essentially represented the interests of the private fee for service medical practitioner and has steadily resisted any form of socialized medicine. Consequently, there has been little fostering of medical education that deals with social needs and how medicine might help improve them. Only reluctantly and tardily has the AMA admitted that medical care is a right for all. Rather than adopt a resolution at its annual meeting in 1973 which would call for the recognition of the "right to medical care" the House of Delegates instead reaffirmed its "existing policy" which was not clearly stated. The record states: "It is the right of every citizen to have access to adequate medical care, but it is the responsibility of the citizen or of society to seek it. The American Medical Association will use all means at its disposal in an endeavor to make adequate medical care available to meet the needs of each person. In the spirit of inheritance of the Oath of Hippocrates, *the AMA reaffirms its obligation to humanity.*"[7] (Italics mine.) What the AMA was "reaffirming" was not the right of every citizen to medical care but rather its traditional obligation to humanity. But they had admitted that access to health care was a right.

During the AMA's golden age there was a great deal of public health promotion and service to society but since the great takeover by the conservatives in 1920, there has been much wind but little rain. Certainly, the deliberate creation of a physician shortage does not promote the public health or serve society. Many more examples can be cited. For example, the AMA has steadily maintained that socialized medical programs are unnecessary largely because American medicine has always provided adequate care without charge for those in need. This is a ridiculous assertion to anyone familiar with the American medical scene and certainly was obvious to the federal legislators who enacted the Medicare-Medicaid laws of 1965, a piece of legislation which the AMA stoutly resisted. Closely allied to an obvious gross inequality of medical services in this country is the problem of physician shortage and/or maldistribution. Yet for years the AMA maintained there was no shortage; it was only a "maldistribution." Not until recently has the AMA supported a drive for more physicians and other health personnel.

The medical profession has always had a number of good men who provided free care to those in need, but there is no reason for believing that they are more than a minority. Paradoxically, now that socialized medicine is a reality, some physicians have refused to participate, saying that the fee schedule is too low, or the payments are too slow.[8] Yet many of these would be the same physicians the AMA claimed were formerly providing free care to the needy. Although I know a few physicians who continue to provide free care to Medicaid-eligible patients rather than go through the paperwork involved in submitting claims for services, I don't think this is common. It is more likely that much of the alleged free care was simply not given in the "good old days." What does emerge as common is the growing practice of fraud and abuse of the Medicare-Medicaid programs by many of the same physicians who originally opposed them. Yet the AMA has insisted there are only a few offenders and that the organization will weed them out; a statement I am still waiting to see implemented.

Public health? There is a long and shocking list of public health programs which the AMA has in fact opposed. It has at various times resisted federally sponsored programs of maternal and child health, crippled children's services, and child welfare despite the fact that in 1975 the United States still ranked fifteenth on the list of countries with the worlds lowest infant mortality figures. The AMA has also opposed free immunization programs, and it is customary in many areas to require those wishing such immunizations from public health clinics to first obtain a release from their private physician. Yet in 1977 five million children were not immunized against six of the common and crippling diseases of childhood for which there are safe and effectives vaccines.[9] The AMA in the past has fought federally subsidized programs of medical examinations for school children, even though such screening has uncovered many remedial defects, especially among the poor.

Service to society? The AMA has resisted Social Security benefits for the totally disabled and extension of health-care benefits for veterans. The AMA had opposed group practices and especially prepaid health care plans until 1943, when it was successfully sued by the United States for monopolistic activity in the health-care field. The title of that action, *The United States* v *the American Medical Association* is indicative of an adversary position that has actually existed for many years; one in which the vested interests of organized medicine were inimical to the best health-care interests of the American public.

To be sure, there have been changes in recent years. The AMA now supports the Medicare-Medicaid programs while reserving the right "to oppose specific statutory or regulatory requirements in the program." In 1976 the AMA voted in favor of a national health insurance plan which some of the hard-liners regarded as treason. On closer examination, however, the AMA was supporting a national plan which would retain the present fee-for-service system with a third party insurance corporation providing the reimbursement. Such a plan would differ little from the current social medicine programs with the same potential for fraud and abuse. The AMA has recognized that federally funded neighborhood health centers, which care for some four million medically needy in this country, "have served a need by providing health care in areas that previously had little or none available and accessible."

The AMA now recognizes health maintenance organizations (HMO) and other prepay forms of group practice as part of a "pluralistic approach to health care delivery." Many local medical societies have instituted health maintenance organizations of their own, although the AMA has cautioned that more "experimentation and evaluation" are needed. In terms of physician distribution and supply, the AMA has opposed any form of draft for civilian service, including the undersupplied Indian Health Service, but has not offered anything of substance as an alternative to relieve the physician shortage. The AMA maintains a physician placement service, but I am unaware of any direct effort made by this service to encourage physicians to serve in an underserved area except in what is called "Project USA." The AMA does manage this federally funded program which attempts to secure temporary substitutes for National Health Service Corps (NHSC) or Indian Health physicians who are on leave. NHSC physicians are normally recruited by the U.S. Public Health Service and assigned for a term of two years to sites designated as underserved. The AMA is now calling the NHSC program wasteful and unnecessary and is asking that the program be terminated. Yet without this service many communities will not have a physician.

In other cases the AMA has opposed free medical care to merchant seamen, which has been a long-standing, traditional inducement for service in that body. The AMA opposed the accreditation of nursing homes in this country by the Joint Commission on Accreditation of Hosptials, of which it is a member. In the wake of the national scandal over the shockingly poor conditions in many nursing homes, the AMA reversed it opposition, but the accreditation process is still hampered and not functioning as it should.

The political strength of the AMA is impressive when it opposes legislation or political appointees it considers unfavorable to its interests. In addition to opposing socialized medicine and other liberal medical legislation, the AMA has effectively blocked the appointment of liberal physicians like the late John H. Knowles who was a candidate for the post of assistant secretary of the Department of HEW in 1969. Yet section 10 of the AMA's Principles of Medical Ethics (1957 revision), which was in effect in 1969, clearly states:

The honored ideals of the medical profession imply that the responsibilities of the physician extend not only to the individual, but also to society where these responsibilities deserve his interest and participation in activites which have the purpose of improving both the health and the well-being of the individual and the community.

Even the diluted version of the above found in the 1980 revision of the Principles (see appendix) clearly indicates a responsibility for improving society. The AMA has not adequately dispensed its own lofty prescription.

The AMA has had some rather curious relationships with the drug industry of this country beginning with its infamous annual meeting in 1920 where the hard-core conservatives asked for and got financial help from the industry to support their fight against the liberals. A cozy relationship has been more-or-less the norm since then. Several former AMA officials have moved into the officialdom of the drug industry or its Washington lobby, the Pharmaceutical Manufacturers' Association. The drug industry has provided the major portion of advertising revenues for the *Journal of the A. M. A.*, representing over $11 million dollars annually, and at various times the *Journal* has been accused of protecting the drug industry by permitting less-than-truthful advertising of pharmaceutical products. An interesting example was a full page ad in the *Journal of the AMA* for November 8, 1976 for Preparation H, a proprietary over-the-counter preparation widely touted for the treatment of hemorrhoids. Yet, in a review by medical experts of the claims made for this product, it was concluded that "there is no acceptable evidence that any of these ingredients, alone or combined in Preparation H can reduce inflammation, cure infection, or shrink hemorrhoids."[10] It is evident that much internal strife has been created within the AMA because of this abuse; not all AMA members are happy with this situation.

Things came to a boil after the AMA opposed the passage of the Kefauver-Harris amendments to the Food and Drug Act. These amendments were proposed following the thalidomide disaster of the early 1960s and called for sweeping reform of the way drugs were evaluated in order to assure not only their safety but their efficacy. In the wake of the bad publicity which the AMA received as a result of this opposition, it undertook the publication of a book to be known as *Drug Evaluations*, which was to be an impartial evaluation of the merits of various drugs for various disease conditions. The task was given to its council on drugs, which selected a group of blue-ribbon pharmacologists to head the project. Publication of the completed first edition was delayed so that the Pharmaceutical Manufacturers Association could examine the proofs. The first edition was ultimately published without too many concessions and was regarded as a good and reliable medical reference work.

However, when the second edition was being prepared, the AMA's board of trustees attempted to weaken the entire thrust of the book by removing the phrase "the council does not recommend this drug," when that was the considered opinion of the council. The editorial staff would not accede, and some time later the board of trustees stopped publication of the second edition by abolishing the council on drugs! A third and fourth edition of *Drug Evaluations* have subsequently been published but lacking the incisiveness and guidance of the earlier edition. The average primary care physician needs authoritative help in his daily practice in the choice of safe and effective drugs from among a confusing array. All too often most of his information comes via the drug company representative. Here again is a great unmet need which the AMA failed to meet properly in an apparent conflict of interest. Had the traditional spirit of *philia* prevailed, this could not have happened.

The AMA refused to endorse the Surgeon General's 1964 report linking cancer with smoking although the American Cancer Society and many other concerned groups did so. A few months later, the Tobacco Industry Research Committee announced it was awarding $10 million to the AMA to conduct further research on the effects of smoking. At that time the AMA testified before the Federal Trade Commission against the use of proposed warning statements on cigarette packages as did the tobacco industry. This is a strange case indeed because the evidence linking cancer and other respiratory ailments with smoking came from reputable medical researchers; facts with which the AMA was well aware. However, it was not until five years later in 1969 that the AMA officially opposed smoking, something that, ethically, it should have done much earlier. Early in 1980 the AMA announced a new drive to curb smoking and urges all physicians to stop smoking and ask their patients to stop. Perhaps recent studies which again link smoking to cardio-respiratory disease have caused this renewed concern.

In 1973 the secretary's Commission on Medical Malpractice (Department of HEW) released the results of its study which concluded there was a lot of malpractice litigation in this country simply because there was a lot of malpractice! Predictably the AMA promptly wrote a minority opinion which disagreed with the findings despite some solid evidence that negligence on the part of physicians caused at least 7.5 percent of hospitalized patients to be injured.[11]

When evidence began to accumulate early in the 1970s that there was an excessive amount of surgery in this country with much of it performed by incompetent surgeons, the AMA disagreed. However, the Study on Surgical Services in the United States or SOSSUS, a task force to study this matter made up of representatives from the American College of Surgeons and the American Surgical Association, concluded that there were too many surgeons, some forty thousand of whom were not board-certified, and over whom there was too little control of training or utilization.[12] With a surplus of surgeons there simply is going to be some unnecessary surgery and that basic law of economics has operated to produce much unnecessary surgery in the United States.

Certain union health care plans became alarmed at the rapidly rising costs their plans incurred and began to suspect there was considerable unnecessary surgery being performed. In 1974 a report was published on the results of an experiment conducted among two labor unions. Members who had been advised to have surgery by their physicians were reexamined by board-certified surgeons who found 24 percent of the recommended procedures unwarranted.[13] When the Congressional Subcommittee on Long-term Care quoted this study as a basis for investigating the whole question of unnecessary surgery, the AMA's executive vice-president, Sammons, fired off a peevish letter to the committee calling the study "unsound" and "unscientific." He then noted that a second medical opinion was a poor way to check on indications for surgery, because, after all, "the second surgeon could be wrong, too."

The AMA's Model Constitution referred to at the beginning of this chapter indicated that a physician should be a community leader and be of superior character. Meanwhile the exhortation that a physician should exercise "courteous and open treatment of his brother physician" is one which is neglected in practice by the AMA. Physicians are sometimes treated shamefully by their colleagues for insufficient or wrong reasons, and promotion of trust and good-will among physicians is an important and neglected function of organized medicine.

We know that the AMA adopted Percival's *Medical Ethics* virtually intact at its first annual meeting in 1847. This code was the norm for American and British medical ethics for many years and echoes of Percival can still be heard in the language of the current Principles of Medical Ethics of the AMA. However, the earlier codified approach could not cover every conceivable situation and so invited abuse. Furthermore, legalistic abuse was easy; one could scrupulously follow the letter of the code and avoid the spirit. For example, one could avoid splitting fees but do unnecessary surgery since that was not specifically forbidden. Also, much space in the early codes was devoted to medical etiquette as well as the more substantive issues so that the whole intent of medical ethics has been much misunderstood.

Although in 1957 the AMA abandoned the codified approach and now uses general ethical principles (with many annotations), there is still too much attention to specifics such as executive physical examinations, social calls on another physician's patient, secret remedies, disposition of drug samples, and so on, and not enough discussion of true ethical principles and general guidelines prepared in the light of the Hippocratic legacy. There is, in short, too much preoccupation in the annotations of the Principles of Medical Ethics with the commercial side of medicine and matters dealing with etiquette. Small wonder my dental friend was confused as to the true meaning of medical ethics.

In 1980, as noted previously, the Principles were reduced from ten to seven, but there has been some weakening or elimination of important clauses of the 1957 version. These changes were reported to have been made with the intent of "modernizing the language, eliminating the reference to gender, and reaching an appropriate stance between professional principles and contemporary society." The article reporting this was contained in the *American Medical News* of August 18, 1980, and went on to note that the AMA's legal counsel had urged changes in the 1957 version (Section 3) because of outstanding chiropractic lawsuits, and Section 5 was interpreted by the Federal Trade Commission as forbidding advertising. However, as one reads through the 1957 and 1980 versions of the Principles it is clear that they have been weakened in many respects, including the social and service-first responsibilities of the physician. It appears that threats of legal action which prompted the revision may have provided a convenient opportunity for the commercial interests in the AMA to effect other changes.

Another criticism of the AMA's treatment of ethics is that the bulk of this work is delegated to the lawyers in the Judicial Council and involves too few physicians. The 1980 revision of the Principles of Ethics did involve some physicians but they were members of an ad hoc committee. Medical ethics is hardly an ad hoc affair and should involve a standing committee with some power to legislate and discipline. An important traditional function has been slighted for too long a time by the country's principal medical organization.

The AMA has stated that one of its purposes is to develop methods "that will moderate the costs of good medical and health care," a position that has as yet produced little effect. On closer examination, this effort seems to have largely taken the form of advice to the member physicians to help contain health costs; advice that seems generally ignored. Since 1961 one estimate has said that physicians' incomes have tripled; if true, this has greatly exceeded the rise in other cost-of-living indices. The total percent of the Gross National Product spent on health care has steadily risen and is now touching 10 percent, a figure that exceeds the national defense budget (1979).

Many major industries in this country are faced with shrinking profits due largely to rapidly increasing costs of their employee health care plans. For example, General Motors paid out $825 million for health expenses during their 1976 model year, thus making Blue Cross and Blue Shield their largest supplier.[14] The general reaction of industry has been to take a hard look at all areas where money could be saved without affecting the quality of the care provided. Many corporations have resorted to utilization review, and to participation in their regional Health Systems Agency (HSA). The HSAs have broad powers of control over the construction or purchase of new health-care facilities and equipment within a designated area and are designed to keep health costs down; thus it would seem prudent for industry to have representation there.

Despite continued denials by the AMA that the medical profession is at fault for escalating costs, a meeting of some of the nation's top-level health-care officials in 1977 placed the blame squarely on the physicians of this country.[15] The consensus among health-care authorities is that cost containment is the ultimate responsibility of the individual physician and that this responsibility has simply not been met. For example, it is only physicians who may admit patients to hospitals and hospitalization costs are a major part of all health care costs. Physicians, it has been said, are not good business persons, and yet the bulk of them in private practice manage to run profitable businesses. It appears that physicians are largely uninformed about the economics of health care and thus unknowing and even uncaring about the costs of health care. It is clear that the average physician is in a very good position to control the cost of health care and has shunned responsibility in this matter. It would have helped if somewhere in the entire professionalization process physicians had been exposed to this important aspect of medical economics. Medical education should implement such an exposure both at the undergraduate and graduate levels; there is nothing to lose and much to be saved.

Some stated purposes of the AMA and their implementation have been reviewed to show the disparity that often exists between the word and the action; at times this disparity amounts to a corporate or group schizophrenia. While the AMA may wishfully think it is a champion of health, ever-responsive to all the medical needs of society in a spirit of selfless devotion, this is obviously not the case. Since 1920 the AMA has represented the vested interests of the private fee-for-service practitioner and supported marketplace medicine—as long as it controlled the major commodities and the vendors. There is no question that at various times AMA policies in the health-care field have been dictated by a ruling oligarchy. Since the structure of the AMA is essentially a federation and not a democracy, it has often been difficult for dissenters to effect changes; however, the major deterrent to change has been apathy on the part of the rank-and-file members. This apathy has resulted in too little input from the members. Still, some needed reforms have been made.

In the 1960s and early 1970s the AMA membership dropped alarmingly. Partly because of this and partly because of internal and external pressures for reform the AMA began to express more liberal ideas and purposes. There are liberals within the AMA who are indeed responsive to societal needs and mindful of traditional obligations but their influence is limited. Although there is a great deal of public and congressional sentiment for reforms in the health care field the AMA has responded only slowly and often with mere tokenism. The main thrust continues to be for the protection of the commercial interests of the entrepreneurial physician.

The AMA has mounted some very curious objections to the "encroachment" of the federal government into the private sector of medicine. During the 1950s, when it was battling proposed legislation for socialized medicine, it directed a huge and expensive campaign to the American public while maintaining a vigorous lobby in Congress. The country was flooded with propaganda pieces, many of which featured a reproduction of a popular Victorian painting of a physician at the bedside, anxiously watching his patient. The caption read: "Let's keep politics out of this picture," which was curious indeed, since the full political power of the AMA was represented by the same piece!

There have been other curious examples of cloudy AMA thinking. Hallowed in the AMA book of Holy Writ is the commandment to preserve the one-to-one patient-doctor relationship and that nothing or no one must intrude into that relationship. Thus the AMA has declared that any socialized medical program "must leave the doctor free to practice in the way he thinks best."[16] This declaration is certainly at odds with any type of peer review or professional control which would provide educational or disciplinary correction to an erring physician and presumably would render the suspension of an impaired physician difficult. Yet, the Principles of Ethics clearly state that a physician must expose deviant physicians. Clearly there are exceptions to the inviolate nature of the patient-doctor model. Also, unanswered is the question of the physician's responsibility to a group or community, for example, in matters affecting the public health and welfare.

A corollary of the first commandment is that the patient must be free to choose his physician. Actually, the armed forces have had socialized medicine of good quality for a very long time; in that system there is little choice of one's physician. The principle of free choice is desirable, but it is not essential to quality care; indeed, such choice may result in poor or dangerous care, for what does the average citizen know about how to choose a competent physician? The AMA carries this freedom-of-choice axiom to absurdity, while historically it has allowed little choice to the physicians of this country in certain matters. Until fairly recently, for example, if a physician was not a member of the local medical society he was generally denied hospital staff privileges—the hospital was a virtually closed shop.

The AMA sanctification of the doctor-patient relationship is either delusional thinking or a smoke screen behind which the *status quo* of private medicine may be preserved. In any event, the relationship itself, along with its corollaries, is not the ultimate criterion of good medical care. A better argument would be for the freedom of the physician to exercise his professional judgment and autonomy while agreeing that his conduct of any given case may be reviewed at some point by a panel of his peers. Such agreement constitutes the traditional spoke of responsibility which must always be coupled with professional autonomy; there is no other safe way.

In the light of the symbolic ethical wheel described earlier, I propose that medical organizations have the same obligation to follow the ethical traditions of the medical profession as does an individual physician. They have a clear responsibility for helping to promote the general welfare and public health in the light of a service tradition which has its roots in *philia* toward one's fellow man. This important tradition of service has been neglected in favor of economic interests which have put the professional cart before the horse.

One final thought: medical organizations in general and the AMA in particular have an important function in protecting the medical profession against *unwarranted* governmental controls. Lay control of medicine is fraught with peril; one of the most valid criticisms against the British National Health Service is the increasing control of the system by a bureaucratic and bungling laity. This has caused much waste, inefficiency, and a depressing effect on the morale of physicians. Our own Congress, in its eagerness to limit the excesses of the medical profession, could enact legislation which would seriously harm the quality of medical care in this country and make the price intolerable. Medical organizations should collaborate closely with the lawmakers while maintaining vigilance against arbitrary governmental controls. Since many physicians are highly individualistic, medical organizations have the potential for converting individualism into needed collective thought and action for collaboration and protection. We need medical organizations to curb the excesses of our lawmakers in the medical field; meanwhile, both our houses could stand some improvement.

While the AMA has done many laudable things, it lacks the public image it has tried to ascribe to itself of honest and faithful service to the public. In 1954 an article in the *Yale Law Review* had this to say about the AMA:

No other voluntary association commands such power within its area of interest.... It holds a position of authority over the individual doctor, wields a determining voice in medical education, controls the conditions of practice, and occupies a unique position of influence in shaping government health policies. Despite the dangers inherent in such a concentration of power, no interest group enjoys more freedom from federal control than organized medicine.[17]

Since 1954 the AMA has lost some of its absolute power, but it is still a force with which to reckon, and it is this older image that stirs the public and its lawmakers for more controls. While the AMA appears to have a lower profile and be much more conciliatory today, largely because of unfavorable publicity, there is little reason for thinking its basic positions have changed.

On reviewing this chapter, I have the same feelings of regret and anguish for the AMA that one would have toward an old acquaintance who came from a good family with a long tradition of serving humanity in philial love, who had the education and other requisites with which to carry on the family tradition, but who, after a few years of useful and devoted service, threw it all away in favor of self-serving. The story of the AMA is thus a tragedy, a montage of opportunities met and lost, of public service, of self service, of self grandizement and delusion, of wrong goals, and of needed reforms. In the eyes of many the AMA is more a trade union than an ethical professional organization and there is much accuracy in this perception.[18] Will *philia* ever prevail in organized medicine?

_____

CHAPTER 5

MARKETPLACE MEDICINE AND PATIENT EXPLOITATION

The preceding chapter demonstrates the split personality of the AMA in this century—a crazy quilt of working for ethical ideals and public welfare juxtaposed with all the power tactics of a labor union for maintaining vested commercial concerns. Why this confused and inconsistent record? On closer scrutiny the record is not as confused as it may seem. Since 1920 the AMA has supported ethical issues which it could afford or were of little consequence or when such programs did not constitute a threat to its economic welfare. In essence the AMA has supported marketplace medicine and insisted on almost absolute freedom of the physician to do as he pleased without "outside" interference.

Herein lie the roots for many inequalities in our health-care system and exploitation of the patient; the entrenched fee-for-service or marketplace basis of American medicine simply cannot work in the best interests of the patient.[1] Fee-for-service simply causes abuses similar to that of the piecework system in a factory; a practice largely abandoned because the reward incentive to turn out many finished pieces caused shoddy work. There is ample evidence that too many medical providers have used the piecework approach to push great numbers of patients through their offices and clinics daily with only the briefest contact with a physician or other medical provider. The entire emphasis is on volume rather than quality, resulting in swollen incomes for many health-care professionals. The U.S. Department of HEW made a point of publishing an annual list of those providers who were paid more than $100,000 by the Medicaid program, but the AMA ultimately blocked further publication by legal action. It has been accurately said that fee-for-service medicine encourages care of the sick more than health maintenance. Does this make sense? The Hippocratic legacy tells us that people should be kept healthy rather than exploited when sick.

The Medicaid program, as well as many insurance programs, has encouraged the same abuse by rendering payment only for care of the sick. In recent years there has been some changes in the direction of early or preventive services, but much more reform is needed. The so-called "Medicaid mills" problem, where high numbers of patients are pushed through a medical facility strictly for profit, has been investigated several times, but so far little reform has resulted. Meanwhile, patients and taxpayers continued to be victimized at the cost of lives, health, and dollars.

In 1976 the media carried a statement by the White House Council on Wage and Price Stability stating that one reason for the tripling of health costs in the past ten years was "the medical profession has monopoly-like control over services and fees."[2] There is just too much evidence of abuses of these Medicaid and insurance programs. At the same time organized medicine repeatedly denies that this is so.[3] It is as if the AMA could not bring itself to believe that any of its members could be motivated by greed or be guilty of fraud and substandard medical care. Physicians are as human and as subject to temptation as anyone else; this is why we have checks and balances such as hospital peer review committees, Professional Standards Review Organizations (PSROs), and disciplinary mechanisms to minimize poor medical care, fraud, or both. The disciplinary tradition demands that organized medicine wage an all-out attack on excesses of this type and stop denying the evidence; token efforts will only prolong the excesses. The public and the third-party carriers have had enough.

It follows that we must take a hard look at fee-for-service or marketplace medicine and ask ourselves if more optimal alternatives might be available. Marketplace medicine is inescapably bound up with patient exploitation and the risk of causing harm simply because there is always the stong scent of money to tempt the physician. When fees are charged for every office visit, every procedure, and every injection, there are always physicians who will give more than is needed, and there are those who will rationalize that such medical care is for the good of the patient. There are some strong-principled physicians who can withstand temptation, but the point is, should they have to undergo such strains? Is there a better way? It may be more feasible to change the system of remuneration than to try to alter basic human nature. History must be the ultimate judge, but meanwhile there is increasing evidence that fee-for-service is the culprit for many of the abuses in current medical care.

It is strange that the AMA considers fee-splitting unethical but fiercely champions the fee-for-service system as fundamental to American medicine. Actually, both cause serious excesses and are interrelated. The AMA seems to have missed the rather obvious point that without a fee, there would be no fee to split! George Crile, Jr., a well-qualified and respected surgical consultant, has strongly stated his belief that surgeons should be salary-based rather than charge fees. Fee-splitting is common in surgical circles for several reasons; the fees are high, the surgeons are numerous, and referrals are hard to get—so many surgeons share the referring physician. Crile points out that persons subscribing to prepaid health plans, as well as the British health service, have about half the surgery of persons who use the private sector of medicine.[4] Because of his firm stand and his prestige Crile has taken much adverse criticism, but he has held firm while the number of authorities who agree with him are increasing daily. Fee-splitting obviously leads to excessive referrals and unnecessary surgery: fee-for-service can cause needless office visits, prolonged treatments, unnecessary procedures and medications. What other alternatives to the fee basis might minimize this abuse?

Most European physicians are now salaried under government-sponsored health-care plans. Health statistics from these countries are good to excellent, despite criticisms by groups like the AMA who decry government in medicine. Surgical rates are impressively low under these national health services, with no increased mortality or complication rates. Another phenomenon noted by Doctor Crile is that when there is a choice between a simple or radical surgical procedure for the same condition, it is the economic factor which often determines which is done. The U.S. is virtually the last country to continue to favor radical mastectomy for breast cancer over the simple method despite ample evidence that outcomes are similar. In Spain Crile was told that the radical procedure is done mostly on private patients, while the simple procedure is the choice in the social security hospitals. The radical procedure simply commands a higher fee but does not produce superior results. It is also more disfiguring.

Despite marked opposition by the AMA to a required second opinion for surgery, it appears the principle is here to stay. Although this opposition caused the U.S. Department of HEW to back away from making this a requirement, it is now calling for voluntary second opinions in the medical programs it funds, and the idea is growing in popularity with the public. At least one state Medicaid program has ordered second surgeon opinions for selected types of surgery over a three-year period to check the effect on costs. Such studies are needed; if they are well-conducted and confirm results of earlier studies, then spokesmen like Crile will be further vindicated.

How do salaried physicians feel about their mode of remuneration? One study conducted among American physicians in private practice and British physicians in the National Health Service showed a higher degree of patient-centered service orientation among the British doctors. The Britons also expressed satisfaction with their salaried status; especially their freedom from collecting fees and their ability to practice according to the needs of the patient without worrying about his financial status; similar sentiments have been echoed by military physicians in this country. However, the American doctors in the study stressed the freedom they enjoyed under the marketplace system and the competitive aspects of working in a free market. The conclusion of this research was that British physicians manifested higher degrees of professionalism especially with respect to the important features of service orientation.[5]

One might conclude that the salaried basis offers a better way to practice medicine and avoids the monetary temptations of fee-for-service practice. However, critics of the salaried approach have asserted that physicians paid by salary are less productive, neglect patients, and shirk their responsibilities. I was unable to find a shred of evidence to support such allegations. There are thousands of salaried physicians in this country working for industry, the military, in group practices and prepaid health-care plans who like their work, practice good medicine, and produce good results. Furthermore, salaried physicians are just as obligated to follow the ethical traditions of service and peer review as their brethren in private practice.

The free-market form of medical practice suffers another serious defect: it is tightly geared to a crisis or episodic type of care because it does not encourage a preventive approach. When you must pay for preventive measures, they are less apt to be utilized. When you're sick enough or injured, you see the doctor, and in between you simply stay away. One of the reasons preventive or "prospective" medicine is hard to teach in medical schools and residency programs is because the students and residents quickly learn that the public, quite literally, won't buy it. Another and equally important reason is that medical students and young physicians in training quickly note that few of their teachers or practicing physicians actually do much in the way of preventive care. That which medical students perceive as hypocrisy they understandably ignore as unimportant. One of the defects in earlier Blue Cross-Blue Shield plans was the lack of coverage for diagnostic and preventive services. This led to the practice of hospitalizing patients for such services under the guise of a spurious medical diagnosis so that the charges would be covered. Finally, the "Blues" caught on and made provision for some ambulatory preventive and diagnostic services. Although there has been some limited increase in the use of preventive services, these are nowhere near optimal utilization.

Some years ago an experiment was carried out by the California Medicaid program to determine the effect of requiring a modest copayment charge (a fee charged the patient) on the utilization of certain clinical services. The most significant finding was a drop in use of the preventive services such as immunization clinics for children.[6] Even a small fee served as a deterrent to the poor who used these health services, largely because they did not perceive preventive services as important. This finding certainly poses a challenge to a program of health education for the public, especially the poor.

Education of the patient regarding the advantages and availability of diagnostic and preventive services is also necessary when they are provided by insurance or prepaid health plans. The negative marketplace attitude toward preventive medicine is one of the reasons that public health clinics offer preventive services without charge. But the "free-market" system does not give up easily; in some localities patients desiring free immunizations must pass a means test for eligibility or get a statement of permission from a private physician! Even when such measures are not necessary, there is some reluctance to attend public health clinics since it is associated with medical care for the poor.

Thus, fee-for-service goes hand-in-hand with the notion that most people should be able to afford medical care. Poverty is a form of disgrace, and the Protestant work ethic demands productivity from all except the most obvious of handicapped persons. To go to free clinics, to be on public assistance programs, to have a Medicaid card is to be smeared with the tar of being a "welfare patient." Despite efforts of the federal and some state governments to provide equal treatment for all, this country is still imbued with the "welfare" or "poor-house" mentality which couples a grudging giving with a bare toleration of these second-class citizens.

Medicaid patients covered under Title XIX of the Social Security Act have the bulk of physicians' fees paid by combined state and federal funds, usually up to 75 percent of the usual and customary fees for a given physician. However, there are some physicians who will not accept Medicaid patients and others may treat them poorly. Patients have been scolded by their physicians because the doctor was not receiving payments promptly enough from the state agency. Other patients are reprimanded for using the emergency rooms for nonemergency medical reasons, a practice certainly not limited to the poor. However, very few private patients are ever subjected to such cavalier treatment.

The high-volume Medicaid mills previously described simply cannot provide quality care with such superficial methods. Furthermore, when poor patients are treated in a patronizing or demeaning manner, many of them respond by not utilizing the services for which they are eligible. A few find the money to pay the doctor's fee rather than suffer the indignity of being a "welfare" patient, but more often the health-care service is underutilized. As a result poor health is still associated with poverty. The fee-for-service system thus discriminates against the poor despite the intent of Social Security legislation to provide them with needed health care on an equal and dignified basis. It is also true that under the marketplace system physicians concentrate in the wealthier geographical areas, which further deprives the poor of access to health-care facilities. Although access to medical care been pronounced as a right for all, this principle is still imperfectly realized under the economics of marketplace medicine—a state of affairs which is counter to medicine's traditional service ethic.

Also, the Hippocratic legacy requires that physicians exercise *philia* toward the disadvantaged, just as did the early Christians. Health-care professionals are effective moulders of public opinion, especially when their traditional role is credible or visible to the public. Hence, if physicians fulfill the *philia* legacy in their attitudes toward the poor, their work will not only be more enjoyable, they can change some of the negative attitudes toward the poor held by society in general. It is especially easy for physicians to fall into the trap of contrasting the life-styles of the poor with their own. Many physicians perceive the poor as "freeloaders," or cheaters, and lazy. This perception is probably generated by the need for physicians to be hard workers and achievement oriented. Some physicians seem to have forgotten that all people are not alike in their abilities and motivations. In orienting medical students in social medicine we remind them that they should avoid being judgmental about the poor with whom they work, and that the poor and disadvantaged are just as desirous of climbing up the social scale as anyone else. The fact that many physicians needed financial and moral support during their long years of training should make them more sensitive to the similar needs of others but sometimes this has the opposite effect.

An alternative to the present system of medical care is some form of publicly funded health-care system for everyone. Present medical care provided under the Social Security Act should utilize full-time salaried physicians who would have free access to medical specialists as needed. The experience of many clinics for the indigent who use part-time salaried physicians has not been good; many of these physicians have part-time private practices as well, and there is a built-in conflict between the needs of the clinic and those of the private practice, and normally the needs of the fee-for-service or private patients triumph. However, the real reform in health care must come in the attitude of both those who provide medical services and those who administer the public plans, a reform which will not be possible without *philia*.

CHAPTER 6

THE ETHICS OF PROFESSIONAL COMPETENCE

Constant concern for the ensuring of professional competence is a primary function of medical organizations and is one of the pillars of our ethical tradition. Moreover, competence must be a shared responsibility of the entire medical fraternity. The Principles of Medical Ethics of the AMA, Section 4, unequivocally state that physicians should safeguard the public and themselves against physicians deficient in moral character or professional competence.

A caveat is needed here concerning the word "competence," one of the four spokes in our allegorical wheel. The competence of a physician is difficult to define and judge. Experts have wrestled with the problem of how to measure competence, but no fully satisfactory method has been devised. There is general agreement that it is composed of knowledge, judgment, technical and manual skills, recognition of one's limitations, and personality. This last item may surprise some, and yet it is a fact that a physician perceived by the patient as warm, friendly, and outgoing is usually regarded as being interested in his patient and may effect a cure or beneficial therapeutic response where other colder physicians have failed. One must apparently like his physician for an optimal therapeutic relationship to be possible.

A familiar poser in our culture runs something like this: "Would you rather be treated by a personable, friendly physician who may not be the most knowledgeable or by a highly skilled and knowledgeable one who appears withdrawn and cool?" One usually hears varied answers to this question but often someone says, "Must these qualities be mutually exclusive?" Of course not; the real point is that the personality of the physician is an important factor in that complex quality we call competence, and this is one of the factors that constitutes the *art* of medicine. However, the real foundation of the art is *philia*, and the patient who senses *philia* from his physician has already made an important step toward recovery.

How then is it possible to ensure competence? At the present time the best that can be done is to assure certain minimal standards which a competent physician should possess. Nothing thus far devised can *guarantee* competence but rather only attest to a certain probability for it. Hence one may establish minimum standards for education, certification, and licensure or may also require peer review and periodic standards for recertification or relicensure. Finally, there are disciplinary methods for assuring these standards, and there is the growing market force known as consumerism.

Educational standards and methods are the backbone of any approach to the acquisition and maintenance of competence. Organized medicine, the specialty boards, and the medical colleges have primary responsibility in this field, which includes the medical school years, the formal postgraduate training, and continuing education for the practicing physician. The medical licensure boards and the teaching hospitals have obvious responsibilities.

The Coordinating Council on Medical Education (CCME) has existed since 1972 and is comprised of members from five parent organizations as described in chapter 4. CCME is charged with the responsibility of recommending policies to all five parent groups concerning accreditation of both undergraduate and graduate medical education and is considered to have broad responsibilities in the review of all matters affecting medical education. Its record to date has been impressive, and there are many reasons for hoping CCME will help set minimum standards for medical education at all three levels in this country. This will establish one parameter for competence at all levels.

Our medical schools must provide students with a sound background for eventual competence in the practice of medicine. Important as this is, it may be even less critical than the selection process for medical school admission. Present selection methods must be critically examined and revised and innovative methods must be employed if we are to have the best candidates from which to fashion competent physicians. Medical schools must pursue this research area vigorously. In addition, better methods must be found for measuring the growth of competence in the medical school and residency training periods as well as the years of practice. This is fully in accord with ethical tradition.

Once a physician has completed formal training years, the state medical licensure boards have been the principal guardians of "competence." This usually means that if a candidate is a graduate of an approved medical school, has no criminal record, and has at least a year of postgraduate training, he is eligible to sit for the board's examination.[1] On successful passing of the examination, the candidate customarily receives a life-time license to practice "medicine and surgery" within the political jurisdiction of that board. If this license is to signify any measure of competence, it would follow that the license must be suspended or revoked if that measure was not maintained. Until just recently, it was only conviction for a felony or gross misconduct which would cause loss or suspension of one's license, and even these actions were limited.[2]

In the past few years there have been growing doubts about the wisdom of granting a life-time franchise to practice medicine, and there is, happily, a reform movement afoot. At this time many states require some form of continuing medical education as a condition of continued licensure, usually in the form of a certain number of hours of approved study per year, and the movement is spreading. There are problems with this approach, but there is also considerable merit. Although it is possible to claim credit for attendance at an educational meeting, one may register and then disappear to the beach, bar, or golf course, or merely doze through the sessions. On the other hand such an exposure may confer a minimum of benefit for a few and cost a great deal for money. Most physicians want to stay abreast of current developments in medicine and will gladly avail themselves of an opportunity, once it is required by law. Such requirements won't of themselves confer competence, but they do make it more difficult to remain substandard. Many older and semiretired physicians have been unable to meet these new educational requirements, and some have voluntarily surrendered their licenses. Painful though this may be, it is in the best interests of society and consistent with our ethical tradition. This movement for relicensure based on required continuing medical education seems likely to spread and may become uniform throughout the country. Although the AMA has opposed such relicensure laws, it has not seriously hampered the trend.

There is also the problem of the so-called "impaired physician," by which is meant any whose competence is diminished by drugs, alcohol, disease, senility, and so on. Only recently has there been a legislative trend to provide medical boards with what has been termed "sick-doctor" powers. Thus, in some states when a physician's professional performance appears to be impaired, the boards so empowered are able to suspend the physician from further practice until the full board may investigate the case and establish the facts. Once an impaired physician is identified and prevented from further practice, the trend has been to recommend a program of therapy or rehabilitation when that seems feasible. These necessary disciplinary actions are corrective rather than punitive and reflect the loving concern for one's colleagues that is an old, if often neglected, tradition of medicine.[3]

There are many horror stories told of injuries and deaths caused by grossly incompetent physicians who continued to practice because no one appeared able or willing to prevent them, and appropriate laws were lacking. Furthermore, medical boards cannot take corrective actions until they have a complaint on which to act. The AMA's Principles of Medical Ethics clearly states: "A physician should expose, without fear or favor, incompetent or corrupt, dishonest, or unethical conduct on the part of members of the profession." (Sec. 4:6) But all too often no complaint is made, or once made, the plaintiff fails to appear or backs down at the hearing. This inertia has given rise to the charge that the medical profession is guilty of a "conspiracy of silence." The change is probably a true one. This reluctance of physicians to testify against one another despite an ethical imperative to do so is both pervasive and difficult to explain.

Concern over the assessment and establishment of competence was one of the primary reasons for the founding of the medical specialty boards. These boards all require minimum standards of medical education and postgraduate training within a given field before the candidate can sit for the qualifying examination. Thus, certification by a specialty board attests to certain standards of education and a demonstration of knowledge by examination but it does not guarantee competence. Other things being equal, a person who possesses board certification can be expected to have a certain amount of expertise within the specialty field not normally present in one who is not certified. Certainly such certification does not guarantee competence in the full sense I have been using here, that amalgam of knowledge, judgment, skill, ethical sensitivity, and personality (to name a few) that makes for a competent physician. There is much disagreement about what constitutes competence but there is general agreement that it is more than technical skill.

Like the state medical license, once specialty certification is acquired, it has been for life. In an effort to avoid the pitfalls of life-time certification, the new American Board of Family Practice requires a definite number of hours of continuing education plus reexamination every six years. Other specialty boards are now headed in the same direction of periodic recertification by the same or similar methods. This is an ethically sound movement.

It is evident by now that all levels of professional education must be involved in the quest for assessing and imparting medical excellence and competence. Peer review is another technique that can be an effective mechanism for curbing incompetence and assessing the quality of medical care. The principle is centuries old and al-Ruhawi first ascribed this practice to the classical Greeks. It is basically a method whereby physicians act as their brother's keeper to keep one another on the proper ethical path. Simply stated, peer review is a survey or audit of the medical care provided by one physician by other physicians having expertise in the field under survey; hence, neurosurgeons would normally review the work of another neurosurgeon, and so on. Society has accepted the fact that physicians are best suited to judge the work of another physician, and this mandate from society to the profession will probably continue as long as physicians do adequate peer review. It is apparent that peer review has not always worked as it should, and when an especially bad example of its failure hits the news media, there is understandably a cry for outside controls.

Health care may be examined or reviewed at three levels, that is, the structure, the process and, the outcome. *Structure* has largely to do with the physicial facilities, equipment, and patient flow. *Process* is the manner in which health-care management is provided and is concerned with how the diagnosis is made, whether further checks or tests should have been made, or whether too many tests and procedures were used; in other words, was the workup appropriate? For each diagnosis the review is concerned with whether appropriate treatment was given and how, and whether follow-up care was provided. When the condition is a reasonably common one, these factors can be compared to a regional average. If hospitalization was provided, was it necessary and was the length of stay appropriate? These are some of the check points which peer review gets into at the process level.

Peer review of *outcome* was popular for a time and is probably the oldest review method, as al Ruhawi indicated. Did the patient get well? Was he unchanged? Did he worsen? Or expire? There is some current interest in reviving methods for assaying outcome once again, especially the effects of health care within a given geographic area, and these can be applied to the results of a single physician as well.[4]

When peer review is provided in a hospital, as it must now be for approval by the Joint Committee for the Accreditation of Hospitals (JCAH), it is generally known as the Quality Assessment Program or QAP. In larger hospitals two or more committees may be involved but usually there is a *utilization review committee* whose function is to review admissions to see if they were indicated and to periodically assess the lengths of stay to see how they compare with normal percentiles for that condition. The attending physician is contacted to explain any deviations. Laymen or allied health personnel may sit on such a committee. The *medical audit committee* is made up of physicians who review the medical records to assess the care provided by a given physician. Laboratory and other diagnostic procedures are checked for relevance along with the general management of the case.

Peer review can be applied to ambulatory care as well, and again it is normally the process that gets examined. Such reviews are often called audits, and they may be external and performed by outside health-care professionals trained in this work, or they may be internal audits and can be simple enough so that office personnel might perform certain checks. For example, when the patient complained of a sore throat, did the physician take a throat culture for the presence of beta hemolytic streptococci? Or did he prescribe an antibiotic?

A growing and increasingly potent control force in the health-care field is the consumer movement, or "consumerism." Consumerism is commonly associated with Ralph Nader, who crusaded successfully several years ago against the auto industry for improved safety standards in new cars. Basic to the concept of consumerism is an informed consumer, who is discriminating in his choice of what and when to buy. An informed consumer of health care (formerly known as a patient) is not intimidated by the superhuman image of the physician and will ask intelligent questions about his care and can also evaluate many of the qualifications of a given physician.

A 1976 article in the *New York Times*[5] quotes one authority as saying that an informed group of consumers can be the most powerful force for improving the quality of health care. These informed patients know how and when to choose doctors and what questions to ask in order to receive adequate preventive care, proper diagnosis and treatment of an illness, and how to find out if surgery is needed. The article contained a detailed suggestion list which consumers should use for choosing competent physicians, including how to "decode" the directory of physicians published by the AMA! Actually, local public interest groups have compiled physician directories in some 30 communities, the *Times* continued, and one should contact the Health Research Group, 2000 P Street N.W., Washington, D.C. 20036, to find out if a directory is available for a given area. The article concludes that informed patients could do more to remove the estimated sixteen thousand physicians totally unfit to practice than could the traditional regulatory mechanisms. Another active consumer group is the Center for Medical Consumers and Health Care Information, Inc. at 410 East 62nd Street, New York, N.Y. 10021.

We have looked at several ways of approaching the problem of assuring competence and have seen that these methods are largely concerned with establishing minimum standards of performance with some powers of enforcement or discipline for maintaining such standards. Once again, discipline is a traditional hallmark of the profession used to assure certain levels of conduct and performace that dates from the guild period. Before assessing how well discipline works in medicine, it will be necessary to review some of the traditional disciplinary mechanisms.

The usual disciplinary actions have been conducted by three groups: the medical society, the hospital staff, and the state medical licensing board.

Medical societies have limited powers of discipline against an offending member physician; the principal methods are censure, suspension, or expulsion from the society. However many physicians do not belong to medical societies. In the "good old Fishbein era," virtually every physician had to be a member of a medical society in order to have hospital privileges; and loss of society membership, threatened or actual, was tantamount to professional suicide. Even though medical societies no longer have such control over practice conditions, the ignominy of being disciplined by one's peers can be a reasonably effective method against some physicians. Still, medical societies do function at the grass-roots level and could be very effective as initiators of actions that could be referred to higher levels if they could not be handled locally. Undoubtedly, many cases involving misconduct charges could be handled at the local level, but this has not been the norm; medical societies have been conspicuously inactive in disciplinary functions.

The hospital medical staff is in a better position to judge a physician's performance than the medical society since it has peer review committees and access to medical records that the society lacks. However, the committees must work well and report deviations from accepted standards to the proper staff authorities for needed disciplinary action. The three methods of censure, suspension, and expulsion from staff membership are also used here. Unfortunately, hospital medical staff action has too often been limited, inappropriately lenient, or aimed at concealing the offenses. In many cases an offending physician is permitted to resign from a hospital staff, which only allows the misconduct or incompetence to be transferred somewhere else; thus, the public is still endangered.

The medical licensing board is more in the nature of a tribunal that must depend on referrals or direct complaints for disciplinary actions. It cannot act unless there is a complaint, and frequently the complainant fails to follow through and appear at a hearing. Medical licensing boards like to have virtually "airtight" cases before they will act, since many guilty physicians have escaped punishment because of legal technicalities. A further problem has been the failure of the various bodies concerned with medical discipline to share information with one another. Not only do the medical societies, hospital staffs, and licensing boards fail to share as they should, but the various state boards have been lax in this regard. Thus, a physician who loses a license in one jurisdiction but who has a license in another state may continue to practice in the second one.

A major problem in medical discipline is the myth cherished by organized medicine that there are only a few deviant physicians and that the profession can handle these disciplinary problems itself. But there are mounting doubts and disagreement about this within the profession itself as witnessed by the following quotations:

The medical profession has always done a good job of regulating itself. In order to assure itself of the right to retain control of its members, the medical profession must be on its guard always against the unethical practitioner or the physician who violates the Medical Practice act.[6]

Does organized medicine adequately discipline unethical physicians? The answer is no.[7]

The first quotation is from the AMA's *Medical Ethics and Discipline Manual* and the second is from an article by Robert C. Derbyshire, a physician and member of the AMA, secretary of the New Mexico Board of Medical Examiners, and a respected authority in the field of medical discipline. Derbyshire has been active for much of his professional life with the Federation of State Medical Boards of the United States and has been prominent in the struggle to improve standards of performance in the medical profession. Derbyshire has reasons for differing with the AMA's opinion that all is well discipline-wise, in fact, the AMA's own *ad hoc* Medical Disciplinary Committee concluded in 1961 that although adequate medical disciplinary mechanisms do exist and are used, the frequency and effectiveness of usage are "less impressive."[8] The committee made several recommendations for improving discipline, and the report was accepted by the AMA.

A recent article in a medical news magazine was captioned "How Well Does Medicine Police Itself?" and continued rhetorically, "Not well enough, as shown by the case of California's Doctor John Nork and a survey of disciplinary actions taken by state boards since 1969."

Nork was an orthopedic surgeon in Sacramento, California, who was found guilty of malpractice in three separate actions.[9] The judge's memorandum of decision on the third case found Nork responsible for negligent surgery and told of at least 50 additional surgical procedures Nork performed that might have been unnecessary or bungled or both. He further charged the surgeon with inducing patients to have surgery with threats, intimidation, and false positive myelograms and afterward of reporting false progress notes and altering the opinions of the medical consultants. The judge further suggested that the medical community had attempted to conceal the malpractice and placed part of the blame on the local medical society and the state board of medical examiners. Equally damaging was Nork's admission that some of the surgery was unnecessary or negligent and that he had been on mood-altering drugs during these periods. The judge in this case also set a legal precedent when he held the hospital corporately responsible for the conduct of its attending staff.

Some other facts deserve emphasis; Nork continued to practice medicine for three months after the judge's decision until his license was finally revoked, even though the board of medical examiners admitted he had been under investigation for two years. Nork had failed the qualifying examinations of the American Board of Orthopedic Surgeons on three occasions, a fact which ought to have been available to the hospital medical staff. The pathologist admitted that Nork had sent specimens from laminectomy surgery (in which the spinal arch is un-roofed to relieve the nerve pressure) that contained *normal* nerve tissue. Normal nerve tissue is rarely, if ever, removed but the pathologist saw no reason to inform any of the medical staff. There had been some irregularities in surgery that had gone unreported to the chief of the department and the judge's memorandum mentioned many opportunities when Nork's competence or medical management might have been challenged.

Even though discipline might not have been called for, the judge noted that a record should have been made of deviations from the normal. It was noted that in only one instance did a reviewing physician suggest that the poor results of Doctor Nork's surgery might be the fault of the surgeon and, in fact, the consultants which Nork had requested for other patients who had suffered poor postoperative results had minimized these findings or falsely ascribed them to the anesthesia, or other causes. Other factors emerged; the hospital had an excellent peer review system but it had failed to detect negligence in this case.

Why had peer review failed to reveal any of Nork's malpractice? One expert testified that peer review assumed that a physician was honest, and the method was not designed to detect fraud. Another assumption was that the medical records were always accurate, but in this case they clearly had been altered and falsified. Other factors emerged: the reviews tended to be ran-

dom, cursory, infrequent, and not critical enough. Too often
they reflected the subjective judgment of the physician reviewer.
The review committee was constantly hampered by lack of time.
One audit was performed during a lunch hour at the hospital
when perhaps 50 laminectomy case records had been selected for
review, but the committee only had time for 18, including several
of Nork's. In one and a half hours, there was insufficient time to
compare nurses' notes with those of the surgeon which would
have shown discrepancies.

It should be noted that California's Board of Medical Examiners operates under the Department of Consumer Affairs and
reflects the high level of consumerism in that state. Nork had
been under investigation for two years by the department, and
the failure of the Board of Medical Examiners to act early was
because they still lacked an air-tight case and not from lack of
interest or motivation. Gathering hard evidence and getting
people to testify is the problem that plagues medical boards more
than any other. An informed consumers' group in Nork's area
might have uncovered his incompetence sooner. Consumerism
had led some states to resort to the issuance of press releases
naming the offending physician and describing his violation. The
consumer movement is believed to be responsible for the
increased disciplinary actions taken against physicians in several
states. The fact that it did not detect Nork does not rule out
consumerism as an effective and growing method for weeding
out incompetents.

All things considered, it was not the failure of the committees
and other safeguards in the hospital which permitted Nork's
incompetence to continue as much as it was the personal default
of his colleagues who were aware of his misconduct and did
nothing. There were many occasions, as the judge noted, when
this tragedy could have been stopped had those knowing physicians followed their professional obligation and sounded the
alarm. A common reason given for failure to act in the past has
been the fear of a retaliatory lawsuit even though this has rarely
been successful. Another reason is said to be the realization of
most every physician that he, too, is capable of erring or has done
so in the past. However, there is a world of difference between an

occasional error and continued incompetence or unprofessional conduct. This kind of self-awareness and resulting hesitation to act is permitting incompetence and misconduct, and as soon as physicians understand this they will be ready to meet their ethical responsibility. It must be done because of the obligation of discipline arising out of *philia*, and when this is a way of life then medicine's credibility will be restored.

There have been increasing warning signs and rumblings that the public will no longer tolerate cover-ups and lack of action. A 1977 article in the *American Medical News* is headed "Disciplinary actions against M.D.'s up sharply." The article attributes this to the passage of many new laws in some 15 states making it mandatory to report professional misconduct. In some cases a physician who fails to report such violations may lose his own license. Several of these states have additional clauses which protect the person reporting from civil liability when the report is made in good faith.[10] Other states are following this trend. Ironically, what could not be accomplished by an ethical obligation is now possible through the legal sanctions which organized medicine has forcibly opposed. If *philia* does not prevail, legislation will.

Some of this new legislation to curb incompetence and misconduct also requires the sharing of information on offending physicians between medical societies, hospital medical staffs, and medical licensing boards. Ultimately, the state boards must share with one another to prevent state hopping by the incompetents. This recommendation to share information was made by the AMA's Disciplinary Committee in 1961 but only recently has any real action materialized.

Local medical societies must become more active in the disciplinary area than previously. This will require vigorous committees that will handle outside complaints by patients as well as complaints by physicians against a colleague. In this way a committee may function as a grand jury and indict a physician on a collective basis rather than having it be the action of an individual physician. Investigations must be done kindly but firmly and fairly and in the spirit of *philia*. Some medical societies are becoming increasingly involved with medical audits of federally funded

medical programs, which has provided them with valuable experience in evaluating physician performance and taking corrective
actions against offenders.

Hospital medical staffs must constantly improve and strength-
en their review committees and mete out effective corrections,
recommendations, and discipline for those who need it. This will
require advice for the treatment of impaired physicians, remedial
education or training for others, and expulsion or limitation of
privileges for some. Again this must always be carried out in the
spirit of *philia*.

Medical licensing boards must have improved functions and
powers with continued, adequate, and guaranteed financing that
does not depend on annual legislative appropriations. Adequate
financing will permit these boards to hire the necessary investi-
gative and legal staffs. Legislatures must give the boards the full
legal powers they need such as "sick doctor" laws and the right to
make a continuing evaluation of physician competence and to
require continuing medical educaton. Finally, these boards need
the support of the entire medical profession, the medical societies, and the hospital medical staffs.

In the light of the obligations of the medical profession in
regard to competence and discipline, it is noteworthy to report
that in 1979 John Nork regained a limited reinstatement of his
medical license in California. He will not be allowed to do surgery
for 15 years and is currently retraining in rehabilitative medicine.
His practice must be supervised by other physicians, and he must
pass tests of psychiatric and clinical competence. He has agreed to
submit to surprise tests on his blood and urine for evidence of
drug or alcohol use. This news is important because it is the story
of a markedly impaired physician who is being rehabilitated by
his colleagues and the state in the finest tradition of brotherhood
and *philia*. More and more states are following this trend of
rehabilitation for sick doctors, and this is a very positive sign of
progress by the profession in self-help and self-discipline.

The Nork case was one of the few sensational ones that occasionally surface and cause considerable furor and possibly overreaction. A similar case was reported in 1975 concerning two
physicians who were twin brothers. Both were qualified gynecol-

ogists on the staff of a New York teaching hospital and had been considered respected authorities in their field.[11] The Marcus twins were found dead in their quarters apparently from an overdose of barbituates. Investigation revealed that the performance of the brothers had been steadily deteriorating for the two years preceding their deaths and that they had actually mutilated some of their patients in surgery. Further investigation disclosed that the hospital administration as well as colleagues had been aware of their erratic behavior and its probable cause; yet no one had acted to offer them help as impaired physicians or curtailed their privileges. Some complaints had been lodged with the local medical society prior to the death of the brothers, but the review process had been too slow; their untimely death and the harm they did to the patients could have been averted by early and determined intervention.

Both the Nork and Marcus cases have spurred legislation to improve reporting of misconduct and disciplinary machinery so that some ultimate good came from both—but what a price! One may well wonder how many cases of incompetence and misconduct with harm or death to patients goes by without receiving corrective action. One unfortunate index is certainly the escalating number of malpractice actions in this country.

An unusual case was reported in 1977 which had a nightmarish quality to it. In 1962 an actress was given a "dietary supplement" of powdered animal bone for dysmenorrhea. Two years later she began to experience progressive fatigue, weakness, dizziness, and irritability. Her health continued to deteriorate, and her career came to an end five years later when she could no longer walk without a cane. In the next several years, the patient consulted some 22 physicians, none of whom made a correct diagnosis and in the course of which she received some 300 X rays. Despairing of ever finding the cause of her illness, she spent several months reading medical books and finally, in 1970, diagnosed her own condition as lead poisoning which was confirmed by a toxicologist.[12] The diagnosis was fairly evident in retrospect.

The bone meal which she had taken until 1968 was found to contain dangerously high levels of lead, and although the patient notified the physician who had prescribed it, he continued to prescribe it for other patients. The patient had reason to believe that some of the other patients of this physician also had lead poisoning from the same source; in fact, one was definitely diagnosed as having lead poisoning. In 1976, some 14 years from the time she started the bone meal supplement, she was diagnosed as having leukemia in addition to the residual lead poisoning. Was it the lead itself, the insecticide residues also found in the meal, or the excessive radiation from the diagnostic X rays which might have caused the leukemia? It seems obvious that incompetence comes in different shades and sizes. It is also curious that no disciplinary action was taken against the physician who prescribed the bone meal and continued to use it for others.

In ideal terms, what is needed for the entire problem of incompetence is not disciplinary nor corrective actions as much as a pervasive mentality of *philia* and professional pride or *philotekne* which expresses itself in a constant search for excellence. To practice preventive medicine, we must seek ever-better candidates for medical school and inculcate the mentality of *philia* and competence throughout the professionalization process and into the practice years as the constant obligation of a physician. A physician reared in such an ambience would find it very difficult to engage in misconduct or let his competence suffer; he would react almost by reflex to prevent this. One would love his profession and its standards as one traditionally loves his parents. Such professionalism is inseparable from *philia* love as Hippocrates understood so well when he said that "where there is love of man, there also is love of the art." Some physicians will always become impaired; this fact renders the detection, reporting, and correcting of incompetence and misconduct totally necessary but only as an adjunct to prevention. Preventing medical incompetence is better than having to treat it; however, failing that, it is certainly time to begin self-healing.

Although the record is not good for self-discipline in medicine, it appears to be improving. Unfortunately, when the courts and lawmakers must intervene, medicine fails in its traditional ethical responsibility. Competence and discipline are two arms of the ethical device which arise from *philia* love and it seems clear that the new laws and guidelines for helping impaired physicians do reflect the design of our ethical symbol. The Hippocratic legacy will work only if it is used and the health care professional who cares about his or her patients will use it well.

CHAPTER 7

SOME UNDERUTILIZED ROLES OF THE PHYSICIAN

Shakespeare once reminded us that the entire world is a stage on which we all play out our roles. Such role playing is an integral and essential part of the performance of the professional person who treads life's stage each day, donning one or more masks in response to the role required by the circumstances of the scene he is playing. One meaning of the word role is "a character assigned or assumed." The nature and the tradition of the medical profession has assigned several important roles to physicians which they have not always assumed. The principal role associated with the modern physician is the one of scientific healer, an identity which needs no elaboration. However, there are several other important, if often unrecognized and neglected, roles of the physician. These are those of priest, advocate, comforter, and steward.

THE PRIESTLY ROLE

By the very nature of his work and tradition, the physician functions in a quasi-priestly role and is often perceived as such by the patient. The physician, though often unaware of the fact, is actually the possessor of a priestly or magical mystique that has a healing quality all of itself. It might also be called a professional mystique, but it seems particularly present in religion and medicine and is coupled with the expectation of the patient or parishioner that the priest or physician can accomplish certain beneficial things not within easy grasp of the average person. The origins of this role and its associated mystiques are lost in antiquity, but the role has been associated with the physician throughout recorded history and appears to have been incorporated into the healing cults of the Pythagoreans, the practitioners of Asklepios, and the medicine men in all primitive cultures.

Studies of primitive cultures, some of which still exist, reveal that the oldest role of the physician was a combined one of priest and healer. A superficial similarity is visible today: the surgical team around the operating table differs little from the priests and assistants around the altar, each garbed in the vestments of the order. A stethoscope dangling from the neck denotes as much mystique and authority as the priestly stole or prophet's mantle; the draping and painting of a site for surgery is a form of unction or chrismation. The priest hearing a confession is not unlike the psychiatrist listening to an outpouring of guilt; the giving and taking of potions not unlike the sacramental bread and wine.

There are other ways a physician, especially the family physician, plays a priestly role. People often turn to the physician as a counselor, just as to a priest. The physician is with the family in times of stress: at birth, illness, injury, and emotional crisis. Also, the physician as priest will not abandon the patient or the family in death; even though it is very difficult for some physicians to deal with death.

Far from minimizing or ignoring the existence of this priestly role, the physician needs to recognize its value in the healing process along with the rituals and "sacraments" of medicine. This effect is undoubtedly psychological, like the placebo effect, but it is a positive factor for enhanced treatment of the patient. The physician, however, must pay a small price for the possession of this power.

No physician should be surprised to know that many patients view him or her as an agent of God or the ultimate source of healing, just as they view their priest, minister, or rabbi as spiritual healers. If the physician is to use this perception in the therapeutic process, he or she must accept the responsibilities which are traditional to a professional person and respect the patient's sensibilities in this regard. Simply stated, if the patient sees the physician as an agent of God then the physician should "act" the part or role and be the good person the patient expects. (It has been said that a drop of humility is needed in the recipe for a superior professional;) the recognition by the physician that he or she is indebted to some power for any healing abilities is an essential part of that humility.

No one should infer from the above that a physician must be a member of some formal religion or profess a certain faith. The quality of being religious is not dependent on such membership or belief. At the same time, in the total or holistic approach to medical care, the physician must be aware of the importance of the religious factor to the patient and must respect the patient's views and values. Many holistic healing centers employ a clergy-man along with a physician and other professionals for multidis-ciplinary diagnosis and treatment.

Advantageous and desirable though the priestly role may be, it is fraught with peril if it leads to the type of excesses described so ably by Thomas Szasz in his *The Theology of Medicine*.[1] He believes that people have often attributed supernatural powers to the clergy with the result that people made slaves of themselves and tyrants of their omnipotent "protectors." A natural alliance then occurs between the clergy and the state. In religion-dominated states, such as Iran in 1980, clergy and government have con-spired to tell people what to believe and how to behave or they face harassment, torture, imprisonment, or death. Szasz likens this to the current conspiracy that exists between many states and the medical establishment, including this country. The most obvious example is the commitment of mental patients, against their will, into institutions for treatment, thus depriving them of their constitutional rights. One of the potential dangers of social-ized medicine is that the state will dictate not only who will be treated, but how and by whom and we who plan for socialized medicine must keep in mind the spectre of Big Brother. Political dissidents are often incarcerated in mental hospitals in Soviet Russia: when the state pays the piper it may call the tune.

The conspiracy between the state and medicine is made easier by the element of paternalism that has long been associated with the healer and which one might view as an abuse of the priestly role. The priestly title of "father" carries the connotation of both a caring parent and one who usurps the decision-making and thinking from his "children," thus keeping them dependent. There are signs that paternalism in the clergy is lessening and the public is growing increasingly restive about paternalism in physicians.

The priestly role is an old and important part in medicine which the superior physician will assume. In so doing, he or she will remember that to fulfill the role adequately one should reflect the good qualities the patient expects in one who transmits healing powers, possibly from a divine source. Properly enacted, the priestly role is not paternalistic but is rather symbolic of an ultimate source of healing and supportive of the other roles of the physician which follow; advocate, comforter, counselor, and steward.

THE ROLE OF ADVOCATE

The word "Advocate" traces its origin to Latin and has at least two meanings; one is "counselor," but the more usual meaning is "one who speaks for or represents another"; thus, in medicine, the physician speaks for or represents the patient rather than acting on his own interests or views. This is easy to see in the legal profession where the attorney is commonly representing the interests of his client. This role, while not quite so visible in medicine is no less important, a point often unappreciated by the medical profession.

Especially in the past, the advocacy role of the physician has often been overshadowed by the paternalistic type of practitioner, who often talked down to his patients and explained little to them about the nature of their disorders or the proposed plan of treatment. Patients were somewhat intimidated, and so they rarely asked questions. That this orientation has changed somewhat in recent decades is not due to any conscious effort on the part of the medical profession but rather to the growth of a much better informed and educated laity insofar as health matters are concerned. The growth of consumerism has also imposed restraints on the free-wheeling of those physicians who "know what is best" for their patients and certainly the malpractice threat has also been a deterrent. Sweet are the uses of adversity at times.

The significance and necessity of the advocacy role is hard for some physicians to grasp. Many physicians are comfortable only when they are firmly in command of the situation by working with accepting and docile patients. Physicians thus oriented are quite possibly insecure without a preponderance of power on their side. This paternalistic type is still with us and is not necessarily an older physician. When this subject was discussed with a number of first-year medical students, many of them forcibly declared that they were obligated to do what *they* felt was best for the patient, in spite of what the patient wished. This reasoning was based on the notion that the patient did not know that was best for him in terms of medical management, which is probably true in many cases. However, these students seemed to have missed the point of their own fallibility and that by pre-empting the rights or wishes of the patient they might be doing him harm.

At least one recognition of this pernicious attitude on the part of physicians (and other health care personnel) is the emergence of a document in 1973 known as the Patient's Bill of Rights. (See Appendix A) This declaration had some far-reaching effects not envisioned by its authors.

An example of harm resulting from a usurpation of the rights and wishes of the patient can be seen in the following fictional account. An unconscious accident victim is brought to the emergency room in a state of shock from blood loss. The attending physician knows the patient to be a member of Jehovah's Witnesses, a religious sect which forbids the use of blood transfusions. The physician could successfully treat the shock with plasma or other blood substitutes without risk to the patient but chooses instead to use whole blood for the "good of the patient." The patient, once recovered, might have serious and lasting difficulties with the notion that his religious scruples had been compromised and that he was contaminated and guilty of sin. In this case, the physician usurped the rights of the patient when it was not medically necessary. Had the patient been conscious and had the transfusion been necessary and permission not been given, the physician would be obligated to respect that refusal or be guilty of assault.

In a similar but less obvious example and one that is fairly common, a physician withholds the truth from a patient who has inoperable cancer and is doomed to die within a reasonably short time. This withholding of truth is either an arbitrary decision or perhaps done in the belief that it is an act of kindness to the patient. Yet this can be an act of cruelty because it may be very important to this man to put his affairs in order and to complete many unfinished items in his life. His anguish will be extreme when he later discovers the truth. Part of the art of medicine is to know when to tell what. If the physician is a true advocate for the patient, he is obligated to respect his wishes and tell the truth on request. This right to the truth is part of the Patient's Bill of Rights.

No physician has an absolute right of dominion over any patient and may not ignore his wishes and rights but rather has a traditional obligation to respect those rights and wishes. When the views of the patient and physician conflict and there is no solution, then the physician must compromise or arrange for the care of the patient by another physician, for the physician has rights as well. In the case of a medical or surgical emergency, the situation can't always be explained to the patient at the time. In these cases and when the patient is a minor or mentally incompetent, the legally responsible next-of-kin must be consulted. Children and the elderly who have lost reasoning powers are segments of our population requiring more than the usual dose of advocacy, for the physician has extra responsibility in such cases. Even if not mature or competent mentally, their rights and wishes must at least be considered.

An ambulatory patient must feel a particular sense of bewilderment in his wanderings as he is shuttled from place to place within the ambulatory clinic jungle of a modern hospital complex. Such a patient has been typically referred to this clinic and that laboratory, yet there is no central control point that can coordinate or follow the course of this patient. Some member of the health team needs to be an advocate for the patient and check periodically on his progress and help to keep him informed and routed back to the proper areas. With the current emergence of so many departments of family practice, one can hope that this problem is self-limiting since the generalist should be the central point of reference. However, some medical centers and hospitals lack family practice clinics or departments, and in these cases some person should be specifically designated as patient advocate. Medical trainees need to be shown the importance of such a role while they are in the teaching hospitals.

Another meaning of the word advocate is "counselor." When life moved more leisurely and physicians had little in the way of specific remedies, there was both the time and the need to talk with patients as persons, offering them advice of all kinds and getting to know them as people. The role of counselor is hard for many modern physicians to fill, often because their practices are busy or because they have no inclination for this type of interaction. This is a tragedy, because many patients visit a physician seeking counsel; when none is forthcoming, they leave disappointed and really not helped very much. To ignore this needed function is to practice fragmented medicine and to foster episodic care and miss much of the joy of being a physician. No physician should be too busy to spend some time interacting with a patient; patients commonly perceive as humanitarian the physician with whom they can easily communicate. With the development of all sorts of physician assistants, more time can be made available to the physician for just this sort of encounter. The interaction skills and counseling ability of a physician are important parts of his armamentarium.

The role of advocate—whether representative or counselor—springs naturally from the tradition of responsibility and *philia* love. When the physician thoroughly understands the crucial importance of the role of advocacy, it will more likely become a vital part of one's style of practice. Patients trust their doctor when they feel that he or she is truly their advocate; such trust is a rich and beautiful thing which any physician will deeply value and not violate. Such trust is one of the great privileges of being a physician and is well-expressed in the AMA Principles of Ethics where it is stated that: "Physicians should merit the confidence of patients entrusted to their care, rendering to each a full measure of service and devotion." (Version of 1957).

Unfortunately, there is a pitfall in this enjoyment of trust, an occupational disease of medicine which I shall call the "adulation disease." Some physicians pass beyond enjoying a merited trust to a state of dependency not only on trust but praise or adulation as well. The problem is that they begin to convert trust into adulation by believing all the compliments they receive or think they receive, when these are often no more than banalities. A drop of humility has been prescribed as the preventive for this disease to effect a self-recognition of one's fallibilities, an awareness which must exist in every truly competent physician.

Once the adulation disease is acquired, it is extremely pernicious, chronic, and destructive. Anything which is perceived by the victim as threatening or reducing that life-supplying stream of adulation is regarded with the same suspicion and hate with which a drug addict would view the threatened loss of his drug supply. Good physicians have succumbed to this disease to the point that they no longer practice good medicine or continue productive relationships with colleagues or patients. Unable to tolerate the loss of a patient who wants to be cared for by another physician, such men refuse to transfer patient records or cooperate in any way, attacking the character of the patient and the new doctor as well. This disorder has been characterized as "professional jealousy," but it is a more profound symptom-complex than mere jealousy. The afflicted physician has forgotten that health management of his patient is the primary goal of medicine and has supplanted the goal with the gratification of his own distorted ego needs. Like the vain but nude emperor, he believes in his own new clothes, and it will take the loving concern and care of his dedicated colleagues to make him see his nakedness. Trust, like alcohol, wisely and moderately enjoyed is a gift, but overindulgence can destroy the best of us.

THE ROLE OF COMFORTER

In this age of the "quick fix" and the miracle cure, it is hard for the public and many of the medical profession alike to accept situations in which there can be no cure and where death or permanent disability is a result. An unknown source tells us that "The role of the physician is to heal sometimes, to relieve often, and to comfort always." Unfortunately, this role of comforter escapes many physicians who view it as a personal failure when they can't prevent death or effect a cure. Terminal situations call for the real art of medicine, yet current medical education is so disease-oriented that physicians forget it is people who have diseases and that everyone needs comforting at times. Several reasons, many of them complex, may help to produce this shortcoming. It is known, for example, that many physicians are drawn to a medical career because they have had some painful encounter with death or disease in a loved one and feel that they must always win in an encounter with either.

Other reasons probably include personal and professional pride and fear of criticism from peers, the family of the patient, nurses, and others. Many physicians react by removing the problem from sight and hence from mind: terminally ill patients are shuttled off to some remote area of the ward where they may often die alone. Professionals such as clergymen who are well acquainted with death and dying and grief in general are usually well-versed in the art of being a comforter. They know that it is an unusual person who wants to die alone, and a primary guideline is that no patient should be forced to endure these final hours by himself.

Since many physicians are unaware of their negative attitudes toward death and incurable or chronic disease, it seems important to deal with this subject at some point in their professionalization. A few years ago the Department of Medicine and Religion of the AMA did some excellent work in this area, bringing together clergy and physicians in joint discussions at both local and national levels. Many physicians learned through these encounters that by developing the art of comforting they no longer felt powerless in these grief situations. In an economy move this program was eliminated as one of the lower priority items. Since the Department of Medicine and Religion no longer exists, this valuable help has been lost. It is to be hoped that medical schools will expand or implement programs in this area aimed at improving the interaction skills of physicians.

One unfortunate result of this inability-to-cure phobia is the generally poor attendance of physicians on nursing-home patients. Many of the patients in nursing homes throughout the country have their care funded through Medicare-Medicaid, and regulations for these programs stipulate that patients be visited on a regular basis by an attending physician and the visits be documented by a progress note. Time after time audits of nursing-home records have revealed virtually total abandonment or neglect of the patients by the physician. When such physicians are candid, they will tell you their reasons for neglect: "I can't stand the smell." "It depresses me to go there, there just isn't anything I can do." This situation was investigated by the Subcommittee on Long Term Care of the U.S. Senate's Special Committee on Aging as a part of their general investigation of nursing-home care in this country. Here are the conclusions from their Supporting Paper No. 3, issued 3 March 1975.

DOCTORS IN NURSING HOMES: THE SHUNNED RESPONSIBILITY

Physicians have shunned their responsibility for nursing home patients. With the exception of a small minority, doctors are infrequent visitors to nursing homes.

Doctors avoid nursing homes for many reasons:

—There is a general shortage of physicians in the United States, estimates vary from 20,000 to 50,000.

—Increasing specialization has left smaller numbers of general practitioners, the physicians most likely to care for nursing home patients.

—Most U.S. medical schools do not emphasize geriatrics to any significant degree in their curricula. This is contrasted with Europe and Scandanavia where geriatrics has developed as a specialty.

—Current regulations for the 16,000 facilities participating in Medicare or Medicaid require comparatively infrequent visits by physicians. The some 7,200 long-term care facilities not participating in these programs have virtually no requirements.

—Medicare and Medicaid regulations constitute a disincentive to physician visits; rules constantly change, pay for nursing home visits is comparatively low, and both programs are bogged down in red tape and endless forms which must be completed.

—Doctors claim that they get too depressed in nursing homes, that nursing homes are unpleasant places to visit, that they are reminded of their own mortality.

—Physicians complain that there are few trained personnel in nursing homes that they can count on to carry out their orders.

—Physicians claim they prefer to spend their limited time tending to the younger members of society; they assert there is little they can do for the infirm elderly. Geriatrics ridicule this premise. Others have described this attitude as the "Marcus Welby Syndrome."

● ● ●

The absence of the physician from the nursing home setting leads to poor patient care. It means placing a heavy burden on the nurses who are asked to perform many diagnostic and therapeutic activities for which they have little training. But there are few registered nurses (65,235) in the Nation's 23,000 nursing homes. These nurses are increasingly tied up with administrative duties such as ordering supplies and filling out Medicare and Medicaid forms. The end result is that unlicensed aides and orderlies with little or no training provide 80 to 90 percent of the care in nursing homes.[2]

In response to such attitudes toward certain segments of our population, the following points need to be said: First, no one was ever promised a rose garden when he or she entered the medical profession, and all candidates from medical school should be told about some of the unpleasant aspects of medical practice. The realities of medical practice; namely, that there are times when patient care is not all sugar and spice, deserve emphasis and reemphasis throughout medical school and graduate training. The challenge is to seek ways to improve patient care. Secondly, physicians must come to grips with their feelings about death and chronic disease, realizing that they reflect to a considerable degree, our cultural attitudes toward the old and chronically afflicted. Thirdly, these physicians have either forgotten or they never learned the importance of the comforter role.

In one area where the physician attendance at nursing homes was exceptionally poor, a physician in the Medicaid program addressed the local medical society, touching on these points and adding that the visit of the physician was one of the few things old people looked forward to. In addition, he reminded them that the nursing staff also felt frustrated and deserted and needed the support and encouragement of the medical staff. Instead of feeling hopeless or powerless, he indicated that they were able to bring some comfort and love into what would otherwise be a pretty lonely and dismal existence. As a result of this discussion, the physicians in that area decided to rotate calls at the nursing home so that one physician made rounds there on a weekly basis and contacted the others as needed. This is an approach based on *philia* and it deserves a trial.

Medical education must explore effective ways to emphasis the importance of this role to students without alienating them. Medical students often rebel and become cynical when they are brought into contact with subjects like chronic disease or preventive medicine or rehabilitative medicine. The method of presenting these subjects must be changed and further, the attitude of the entire medical community must be more positive and supportive of topics like these. To the virtual exclusion of these topics, the bulk of the medical profession is geared to an episodic or crisis brand of medical care popularized in novels and screen plays. Students must somehow learn that the real challenges of medicine lie in the prevention of disease, in keeping patients well, in fostering health education for self-care and in learning and practicing the principles of rehabilitative medicine. These are not only challenges but mandates and the ethical responsibilities of medicine.

A psychiatrist once told me of an experience he would never forget. He was prowling around the grounds of a large state mental hospital and finally, on whim, entered a building he had never visited before. It proved to be filled with some of the most severely retarded patients he had ever seen, and they were being attended by elderly nuns and clergymen who had volunteered their services. He wondered at such unseen and truly devoted service, and as he left the ward he noted a small placard containing a quotation from the Gospel according to Saint Matthew: "Truly, I say to you, as you did it to one of the least of these my brethren, you did it to me."[3] The quotation is from a parable which Jesus related to his disciples, but the meaning is clear enough. Anyone who performs an act of love or kindness to a fellow human is showing his love for God. This is another way of stating the two Great Commandments.

In our Western culture, with at least its nominal allegiance to the Judeo-Christian tradition, it seems clear that the role of comforter has been handed down as an important one for mankind to follow. One of the greatest needs in our individual lives is the therapy of comfort from time to time, yet it appears to be one of the lesser used tools in the physician's armamentarium. It is a prime example of *philia*.

THE ROLE OF STEWARDSHIP

Stewardship is a concept which Christianity embraced, developed, and gave special emphasis, but the role has implications and applications for all of us. The modern word economy traces its origin to the Greek word for steward so that although the original word for steward meant one who was the overseer for the goods or property of another; it also meant one who was a conserver of such goods and managed them wisely. The Christian interpretation of stewardship is that all worldly goods and human life itself are gifts from the Creator to be used or held in trust for a lifetime, that these gifts should be used wisely, and that there will be an accounting of that usage at some future time. Such a concept of stewardship would be close to the conservationist position which views the earth or biosphere as a close system in which man must constantly and carefully plan to avoid reckless depletion of natural resources and to avoid disturbing the national balance of our ecosystem.

Certainly the tradition of the physician calls for the stewardship role, a concept which the training years should reinforce. In this role the physician is a steward of health, a conserver of the gift of life, and should be seeking ways to improve its quality. Just as in the Biblical parable on stewardship, we are expected to return to the originator of the gift more than we received.[4] Ultimately, there will be an accounting of how well the medical profession exercised its stewardship of health to the citizens of this earth. A clear understanding of stewardship principles is a great help in solving specific or more general ethical issues in medicine. True stewardship is love in action; *philia* toward mankind and especially toward those who need the help of the medical profession.

Since physicians deal with human life, it is essential that they define just what it is that makes a life human. It is curious that not too much attention has been paid to such a definition until relatively recently. In 1972, Joseph Fletcher set forth a tentative profile of humanhood consisting of 15 positive criteria and five negative ones, indicating this was only a tentative list to launch a discussion.[5] He invited comment and criticism, which were not long in coming. Based on these responses, he narrowed the criteria to just four in a later article.[6] Most respondents were in agreement that neocortical brain activity was the one essential quality for being human, but that it alone did not constitute humanhood. Others feel that the ability to think is uniquely human and certainly constitutes humanhood in one who is conscious. Yet the single criterion for death on which most would concur is the cessation of brainwave activity, that is, the absence of neocortical function as determined by the electroencephalograph. In the absence of such activity, a physician could *ethically* withdraw all artificial support because humanhood no longer existed.

The second criterion on which many critics agreed was the presence of self-awareness. Fetuses lack such awareness, and it has been held that they may ethically be aborted for sufficient cause because they lack humanhood. However, caution is in order in using this criterion since unconscious patients lack self-awareness, and many of them ultimately recover full humanhood.

At the other end of life's spectrum are the elderly, many of whom lack self-awareness permanently. The elderly who lack self-awareness have usually lost the ability to relate to other humans, the third criterion of humanhood on which there was substantial agreement. With two criteria for humanhood absent one may wonder whether such old people would elect, if they could, to "live" any longer. However, caution is also needed here since certain classes of mental patients lack the ability to relate to others but still retain humanhood.

On the fourth criterion, happiness, there was less agreement since many idiots and animals appear happy. Fletcher contends, and I agree, that the criterion of neocortical function alone necessarily includes all other criteria since none of the others are possible without it. In essence, then, humanhood requires a functioning neocortex in *homo sapiens* which is capable of self awareness, relating to others, thinking, and of achieving happiness. Furthermore, brain death or permanent cessation of neocortical activity is irreversible and may be medically determined whereas the other criteria cannot be absolutely determined. Mere vegetative life cannot be considered human by the above criteria.

The physician as steward of health has a vital responsibility to improve the quality of life just as a good farmer seeks the best environment for his crops and animals. The phrase "quality of life" has been abused and distorted at times, but it is useful nonetheless. No human being should live in misery and poor health, lacking the most basic necessities of life, yet millions of people do live that way on this planet. The steward of health will seek and implement ways to improve the quality of life, especially in the area of health. This means curative and palliative medical care, but it also means more preventive medicine, better public health, and patient education for self-care.

The steward of health also has a role in the allocation of scarce medical resources. For example, there may be one renal dialysis machine for 100 patients who need it to stay alive, but this exceeds the machine's capacity. In such a case who should be dialyzed? Some will say it can only be decided by lot since everyone must have an equal chance; others might say it should be given only to those who possess humanhood with a reasonable chance of recovery. Still others might say that a gifted scientist or renowned jurist should be given priority. The physician, as medical steward, should help to decide each case on its own merits, in the context of *philia*, and in the company of others concerned with the health-care field. Since situation ethics works case by case, no neat formula can be applied, but broad principles may be useful.

A less obvious example is the allocation of health-care personnel to medically underserved areas, a problem sometimes discussed under the heading of "distributive justice." Who, if anyone, should determine such allocations and how? By lottery? Persuasion? Moral obligation? Laws? Again, it seems clear in the light of the Hippocratic legacy that it is the medical profession which should face the problem and help bring about the solution. Certain federally subsidized programs designed to relieve such medical manpower shortages have not worked well and offer no permanent solution. However, medical stewards working closely with government and other concerned organizations, in the spirit of *philia*, could surely supply medical care where it is needed. The responsibility to do so seems plain; now medical stewards must seek out ways.

As conservers of human life concerned with its quality, the physician-steward will promote and prescribe birth control measures to keep our population within the optimal numbers the earth will support. Countries such as India and China are overpopulated; a problem which is taxing these countries and ultimately the world to the breaking point. If, as good stewards, physicians are to attack this global problem they must all be involved and demonstrate their willingness and ability to help poorer nations with their intertwined problems of hunger and overpopulation. There is sound logic in offering food and contraceptives together. No sane farmer would permit his crops to grow so thickly that they would choke out each other so that only a few stunted specimens survived.

In the early days of New England, the colonists learned how to plant corn from the Indians. The ancient formula called for the dropping of five or six seed kernels into each site in the hope that one seed would survive and flourish: "one for the beetle, two for the crow, one to rot and one to grow." The mortality rate for the people of those days was not much better; a woman could count herself lucky if half of her pregnancies resulted in school-age children. Now, with fertilizers and insecticides, we have improved agricultural methods, and we also have public health, a devotion to sanitation, and preventive medical measures, which have greatly lessened our mortality figures, especially in the neonatal or perinatal areas. Yet there are many countries that are lacking such programs, and we must try to help.

Years ago, some well-meaning but uninformed representatives of one of the birth control groups paid a visit to "Papa Doc" Duvalier, long-time dictator of Haiti. They told the doctor that they wished to implement birth control programs in his country. Papa Doc's answer was that there was no need for outside help in this regard, for the naturally high mortality associated with poverty did its own birth controlling.[7] This story may or may not be true but it points to an important principle of ecology; there are natural checks and balances on the numerical increase of any life form. If we remove any of these limiting or controlling factors with improved sanitation, health care, or preventive medicine, then we must be prepared to control population by some other methods. Quality of life applies to the totality of life, not just a portion of it; if we improve human mortality we must hold down the birth rate in some areas. Quantity is directly related to quality after a certain point is reached: since we don't have the instinct for mass self-destruction that certain animal species have when they reach a certain number, we must use better methods now available to us. The steward of health must be aware of the potential dangers in programs designed to modify human ecology; a balance of effects is needed in seeking to improve the human condition.

The word euthanasia literally means "good death" but unfortunately, it has acquired some unsavory connotations and associations which have almost served to make it useless. Here euthanasia and will apply to the mode of providing a good and timely death for those in need. By good is meant a painless and nontraumatic method as contrasted with a painful or hopelessly drawn-out process. If death is not always pleasant, it can be a relatively easy and painless event, and for many it is a relief and release from a burdensome existence. For those who lack self-awareness the event can take place without recognition and would avoid mental anguish for the individual involved.

Part of the problem in talking dispassionately about death is that it is a sinister event for most of us. We inwardly know that no one can avoid it, yet we ignore it as much as possible and try not to discuss it. Seen in its broadest perspective, however, death should be viewed as a natural and desirable part of the life-death continuum or the cycle of life which is seen in all living things. This viewpoint obviously excludes the untimely or the tragic and accidental death and is concerned only with a death which is naturally indicated.

Pet owners frequently take their aged or chronically ill animals to the veterinarian for direct euthanasia or mercy-killing as an act of love to prevent further suffering. The movie cowboy, with tears in his eyes, shoots his horse after it has broken a leg; again as an act of mercy or caring. One can understand the emotions but not the logic of those who say that humans should not be treated the same way, for after all, humans aren't animals. That is true, but as Fletcher and others have pointed out, that vegetative life which remains in a person for whom humanhood has gone is not "human" either. Furthermore, there are those in a terminal condition who want release. Are we to ignore them? Yet the occasional person who performs a merciful act of direct euthanasia is often prosecuted for homicide or manslaughter and sometimes imprisoned.

A common argument against euthanasia is that this is "playing God" since we and not God have decided when someone is to die. We do not apply this argument to suffering animals but are they not also creatures of God? Furthermore, we may twist this argument to say that we should not treat disease nor relieve suffering in humans for would this not be thwarting Divine will by playing God? Hardly so, if God is all merciful and all loving. No, the question is not whether we should play God for it appears that we must. As agents or coworkers of God we have no choice but to make decisions some of which will involve the loving use of euthanasia. If we continue to raise problems by our expanding science and technology then we must be prepared to deal responsibly with them. The real question, then, is how well and responsibly we do play God; this is the central theme of Leroy Augenstein's *Come Let Us Play God*.[8] What is needed is man—come of age—to act responsibly for God in the light of *philia* and stewardship.

The Roman Catholic church supports the principle of indirect euthanasia in that extraordinary means or unusual and heroic support measures may be withdrawn from a patient so that the patient may peacefully die. The terms "ordinary" and "extraordinary" are subject to interpretation. For example, heroic measures for maintaining the life of a 28-year-old father who supports a family may be judged as ordinary, when to apply these same measures to an elderly person with little or no hope of recovery would be judged extraordinary. Other churches have sanctioned the withdrawal of artifical support from a patient for whom there is no possibility of recovery as in irreversible coma or when there is brain death; that is, when humanhood is gone.

I am unaware of any church which sanctions direct euthanasia although some individual theologians have done so. Direct euthanasia requires positive or direct action to cause death such as the giving of a lethal drug, and this is repugnant to some. However, it should be clear that whether the direct or the indirect approach is used, there is only one end in mind; the termination of whatever type of life remains in the patient. Furthermore, the distinction between direct and indirect methods is not always sharp. If the intravenous feeding of a patient is stopped, is that direct or indirect euthanasia? Suppose someone is locked up so that he cannot eat and so starves to death, what would that be? If the first act was done in loving mercy it would be an act of euthanasia surely, but we might quibble about whether it was direct or indirect. In the second act, if it were done with malice aforethought, it would be judged as murder, if malice was absent it might be manslaughter. But it is not euthanasia unless there is a clear-cut reason for the intervention based on the spirit of mercy, of *philia* love. Thus, the motive and the consequences are critical factors. Now, if loving mercy is the essence of euthanasia it can only be a question of time before the direct approach is sanctioned by some church with the courage and clarity of vision to see this act for what it is; the ultimate in *philia* and a distinct act of stewardship.

Doctor Henry Van Dusen and his wife committed suicide in 1975. He was a prominent theologian and former president of Union Theological Seminary, and he and his wife were both members of the Euthanasia Society and advocates of the right of an individual to terminate his or her own life. When faced with debilitating old age and physical suffering, they committed suicide in accordance with a pact they had made. Had direct euthanasia been available to them it is interesting to speculate whether they would have made an application for that route; it seems probable that they would.

In any discussion on euthanasia, in addition to the "playing God" ploy that is brought up, there is usually someone who says,

"But euthanasia is the way the Nazis got started with their mass murders and other atrocities." Such a statement reflects a persistent, unfortunate misconception. The Nazis used the code word "euthanasia" to disguise their program of negative eugenics or killing of those people of so-called *Aryan* origin whose bioracial characteristics were viewed by the Nazis as harmful to the "racial health" of the German *Volk*. The Nazis were not at all interested in true euthanasia as we understand it here: euthanasia requires mercy and love. Furthermore, the program of oppression and extermination of the Jews was never disguised as "euthanasia" and was given an entirely different code name.[9]

It is argued that once euthanasia of any sort is permitted, it will be like the tip of a wedge which, once allowed, will lead to further expansion and finally be used to eliminate anyone deemed undesirable. The wedge argument and its fellow-traveller, the "slippery slope analogy" has proven true only in countries with totalitarian governments. Euthanasia can be expanded and used solely to benefit the person in need and for whom adequate safeguards have been established. It has been legally established that there is a right-to-die in this country which is guaranteed by the language of the Constitution.[10] In the light of this interpretation anyone may refuse any sort of medical treatment even if such refusal will cause death. Surely such refusal amounts to self-euthanasia or slow suicide in many cases, and this is legally permitted. Only in exceptional cases have some courts ordered treatment given, mostly where the patient's exact wishes were unclear.

In the past few years there has been a flurry of interest in right-to-death legislation, sometimes called "natural death acts," to permit the legal use of indirect euthanasia. In 1975 New Jersey made it legally possible to withdraw life support systems under certain conditions, California passed a natural death act in 1976, and by 1979 seven other states have followed suit. Many other states are considering or debating such legislation, and it is possible that natural death acts may become uniform throughout the country. There are many people and groups which oppose such legislation, but it seems clear that there is currently a favorable climate for making right-to-death a specific legal right. An exception was the Maryland legislature, which in 1977 defeated a right-to-death bill on the grounds that it would lead to euthanasia! Notable in these acts is the provision for safeguards such as an ethics committee to approve indirect euthanasia and legal immunity for the physician(s) who actually terminate the support. Other protections for the patient are provided as well.

Long before natural death acts were passed, the Euthanasia Society had fostered the use of an instrument known as a "living will." (See appendix E). This document is executed by a rational person as protection against the time when artificial support might be used to prolong his life; in other words it is a statement of an individual's belief in his right to die. The wording specifically states that extraordinary means for maintaining "life" in the face of hopeless odds shall not be used. Such a document is entirely compatible with the principles of good stewardship, but until the passage of right-to-death acts, these living wills were not legally binding. One hopes that these wills will become uniformly binding in all the states in the same way as the Uniform Anatomical Gift Act.[11]

An example of the need for uniform legislation for the right-to-die is seen in the case of our old people in America. Our cultural norm now is for a small or nuclear family and to avoid having the elderly in our homes. Using what Philip Slater calls the "Toilet Assumption," we flush away, with porcelain and chromium efficiency, our old people or any other "undesirables" into institutions where they are safely hidden from sight and thought.[12] These institutions are little more than warehouses for the living dead, since so many of the elderly quickly deteriorate in such facilities and lose their identity and self-awareness. When this happens, they are often labeled as "senile dementia" and are kept alive in a synthetic environment but are not allowed the mercy of euthanasia. Deserted, forgotten, and unloved, they maintain a nonhuman existence. Before antibiotics, pneumonia was known as "the old man's friend," an insight we seem to have lost, for all too frequently when old people get pneumonia they are given antibiotics and oxygen without their consent. We don't want them in our homes, and we neglect them in institutions, but we won't permit them the right to die which many would welcome. We deny them the dignity of a timely and natural death; we refuse them the mercy and love we commonly extend to animals.

Our society is similarly schizophrenic in regard to infants suffering from severe birth defects or from incurable genetic disease when either of these is serious enough to prevent a normal life or has a progressively downhill course. Children like this are commonly kept alive only by intensive, costly, and ultimately futile care. One recent case of this kind presented at a medical conference is representative of many. The problem was what to do in the further management of an infant with multiple birth defeats. The child was 18 months old and failing to thrive despite all-out efforts by various medical specialists and intensive nursing care. The parents now owed in excess of $50,000 for medical services which they could not pay. In the face of mounting costs and no hope of a normal life or even survival for much longer, some of the medical staff favored the withdrawal of medical support and some did not. The parents had anguished since the birth of the child, alternately between hope and despair for their baby. The cost of the treatment used in vain on this infant could have been used to treat those with better chances for a normal life and for research and prevention of similar tragedies.

Many of the physicians and nurses at the conference were visibly emotional over the issues, which made resolution more difficult. It was the theologian present who did most to clarify the principles involved and recommended withdrawal of support. Although the parents were willing to let this be done, many of the health professionals were opposed to this course of action. Emotionalism had kept medical stewardship at bay, which only increased the suffering of the child and his parents. Could tragedies like this be prevented?

The answer is a qualified "yes"; qualified because although we have reliable test procedures for the detection of carriers of genetic diseases, these tests are purely voluntary and not many couples request them. Once a child is conceived, there are test procedures for detecting a genetically diseased fetus, but again, these are voluntary tests and a sea of controversy surrounds the issue of compulsory screening.

Geneticists have estimated that each one of us now carries from three to ten genes capable of producing a defective fetus. Fortunately, most of these disease-producing genes tend to extinguish themselves and are recessive; meaning that the same disease trait must be present in the genes of both parents' sex cells to produce overt disease or defect in an offspring. Since neither parent in such circumstances displays the overt disease, (a condition known as the carrier state) the only way to limit the possibility of producing a child with the disease in question is to genetically screen both sexual partners. When such matings are not protected by contraception or sterilization, then genetically defective offspring with visible birth defects may result.

Genetic defects can be detected by amniocentesis, a laboratory analysis of the amniotic fluid surrounding the fetus in the mother. Once detected, the issue of whether to abort or not must be raised. If an abortion is not performed (or does not occur spontaneously), then a defective child will be born. Whereas formerly many of these seriously afflicted children died early, medical science now keeps some of them alive to the age where they can procreate, thus increasing the contamination of the human "gene pool." The genetic make-up of any individual is a chance combination of the genetic material randomly drawn from the gene pools of both parents, a process which may be viewed as a genetic lottery. At the point of conception, the lottery is for "keeps," where the winners are those who escape frank genetic disease and can further their chances for having winning children by having themselves genetically screened. To improve the odds of winning we must select ways to improve the wanton reproductive lottery that is now the norm.

If we continue the unchecked pollution of the gene pool by the process outlined above, then it is possible for the human race to ultimately extinguish itself in an apocalypse of genetic defects; a state which has been called "genetic twilight." Some authorities, such as Lappé, now argue that a genetic twilight is only a very remote possibility, whose prevention does not require coercive nor legal modes of control.[13]

To my knowledge, no one has contended that it would be wrong or harmful to reduce or eliminate genetic disease. However, controversy boils regarding the risks and dangers of permitting the present situation to continue unchecked. For example, the only practical method of control prior to conception now is genetic screening of prospective parents. Immediately we encounter the issue of whether such screening should be voluntary or mandatory; there are problems with each. In the voluntary approach, some sexual partners would opt for screening and some would not. If made mandatory, it is obvious that enforcement would be difficult because of the sexual freedom and the great emphasis on individual rights that is current. But let's look at some of the pros and cons of enforced genetic screening commonly used to thwart not only the possibility, however remote, of a genetic twilight but to decrease, however slightly, the number of children born with genetic disease for whom the quality of life may be impaired.

PRO	CON
A child has a right to be born as healthy as possible and might not otherwise elect to be born.	It is a constitutional right of parents to determine the number of children they will bear and what is best for them. To require screening is an invasion of privacy.
Responsible parents do not want to burden society or themselves with defective children and are mindful of the common good.	Detection of a carrier state for a genetic disease may result in discrimination against or stigmatization of the affected person.
Disabled and defective children often end up as wards of the state at a cost of billions of dollars annually. Many of these lack humanhood or a decent quality of life.	Caring for the diseased and disabled is part of our Western cultural heritage.
There are public health concerns for a healthy society. Even if genetic twilight is an unproven theory, who wants to risk testing it?	It is an arrogation of human rights for the state to determine what is genetically desirable and leads to the abuses of eugenics programs like those of Nazi Germany.
Other family members have rights which a defective child may compromise. Psychological effects on the family with such a child may be profoundly adverse.	Since the unborn fetus can't speak for itself, its rights must prevail.

PRO

If we are to limit our population, as appears mandatory, then the quality-of-life issue becomes critical; a smaller population requires a healthier society.

Genetic records can be adequately protected as regards confidentiality.

Children are not chattel of their parents but have rights, including a decent quality of life.

The ultimate concern must be the greatest good for the greatest number: society should not suffer because of irresponsible or thoughtless parents.

CON

There should be no genetic screening unless there is an adequate treatment for that particular disorder.

Genetic twilight is not possible or only theoretically possible.

Most people would prefer not to know that they are carriers of a lethal or harmful genetic disorder and have a right not to know.

Individual rights of parents must be the overriding consideration.

If prospective parents are screened for genetic disease traits and one or more is found, then there are further ethical problems to be faced. "Genetic engineering" or deliberate biochemical manipulation to repair defective genes is theoretically possible but still many years away in practice. Until then, other methods must suffice as society determines. Again, the voluntary decision to have children or not is one option that has only limited application. Voluntary decisions not to have children requires enlightened, conscientious and socially responsible people. Mandatory controls against reproduction pose serious problems for some ethicists and others who would not favor state interference in this area.

We have long had limited laws against the marriage of close relatives; many jurisdictions and churches prohibit first cousin marriages. Taboos against incest are almost universal among primitive cultures, and in both these examples these laws and taboos resulted when it was noted early in our social development that consanguinous matings were more apt to produce defective offspring. Animal breeders are well aware of the dangers of continued inbreeding. The sociobiologists have observed that when unrelated children are reared in close daily contact, as in the Israeli communes, they are unlikely to intermarry: they theorize that some reflex behavior or biofeedback mistakenly identifies one's close companions as family members. In any case, custom, law, and possibly biofeedback have all conspired to limit consanguinous matings and associated risks.

Yet, we have no laws to require genetic screening after the manner of the old laws requiring premarital blood tests for syphillis. A hotly debated exception is the required premarital screening for the sickle cell trait in a few states. Some apologists have called this practice "discriminatory" since the disorder is confined to blacks, and the laws may be repealed. But what responsible parent of any race would want to beget a child with a crippling but preventable disease? If a genetic disease trait should be uncovered by voluntary screening, we have no laws to prevent marriage or childbearing. If a woman who shares a genetic disease trait with her mate becomes pregnant, there are no laws requiring amniocentesis. If tests reveal a genetically diseased fetus, there are no laws to require termination of the pregnancy or to prevent the parents from further begetting of children. Legislation to implement such preventive measures is a political hot potato on which more than one politician has been burned.

There are laws for genetic screening of the newborn for PKU disease (phenylketonuria) as well as the limited laws for sickle cell screening, but there is considerable opposition from many ethicists and others to further required screening. Yet we still have the old laws, civil and religious, against consanguinous matings! Conventional morality appears to be a stronger force at this time than is genetic disease. While many ethicists contend that required genetic screening is unethical, good stewardship would say it is as unethical not to screen. I see the results of genetic disease daily and it hurts to think some of this could have been avoided. At this point, I can agree with John Osmundsen's provocative article that reminds us we are all carriers of genetic disease and that the issues are "troubled by a confusion of ethicists."[14] We need fewer apologists and more clear thinkers equipped to deal with the problems of genetic disease, which remains as much a public health concern as required immunizations for school children.

Even if we had universal genetic screening and other methods for limiting genetic disease, it would still occur to some degree. There will always be those who violate the law, and some genetic disease will defy early detection or diagnosis. But these facts hardly constitute an argument against mandatory screening. Denmark is a country that requires premarital genetic screening with subsequent sterilization of one of the marriage partners should the screen indicate the possibility of a genetically diseased child. Even if we agree that this will only partially control the problem of genetic disease we may also agree that it is a positive step to improve the quality of life. There has been no mass exodus from Denmark, and it appears that the Danes are satisfied with this arrangement. Unfortunately, most of the feeling against mandatory screening in this country is based on emotion rather than logic, with charges of discrimination and genocide raised by minority groups and the general charge made that such required screening violates constitutional rights and is an invasion of privacy. It is curious in all this clamor about individual rights that we do not hear an equal clamor for the individual responsibility that is needed for good citizenship.

The medical steward, by virtue of his training, has more knowledge in this area than the average citizen and hence has a responsibility out of *philia* to acquaint the public with the dangers of genetic disease and the importance of genetic screening. As a conserver of life, concerned with its quality, the health-care professional will work for both voluntary and mandatory screening until the time that we all live in *philia*, responsibly, or until other methods of control are perfected. Furthermore, if medical science is to extend the life of those with serious genetic disorders, then it is prudent, in the light of stewardship, to see that such persons do not propogate their disorder.

But what are we to do if, despite genetic screening, a woman is found to be carrying a genetically defective fetus? Abortion is an emotionally charged issue for many people and because of the intense and bitter debate between those who favor and those who oppose abortion, the issues seem never to be set forth satisfactorily by either camp. How might one approach this problem in the light of sound stewardship and the Hippocratic legacy? First, the basic issue must be identified.

The basic issue in the contemplated abortion of a diseased or defective fetus is a debate over the sanctity of life versus the quality of life. While we cannot predict that a given fetus will be normal or gifted, we can often accurately determine that a fetus is defective and predict the quality of life the child will have, once born. It is counter to good stewardship to permit the birth of a child with serious defects for whom humanhood may be absent or for whom life may be agony. A tour through any of several institutions for the care of such children should be made by anyone who insists on the sanctity of life at all costs. Many of these children are unable to move and totally lack humanhood; they are doomed to lie in a bed and have nutrition literally poured in one end and then cleaned up on the other. In some cases they can neither see nor hear: What kind of a "life" is that? The medical steward is concerned with the sanctity of *humanhood* more than the sanctity of life and wants to assure that anyone possessing humanhood has a decent quality of life. The principles of conservation and *philia* require us to carefully consider the projected kind of life the newborn may have.

Another important consideration is the wishes of the parents in regard to the fate of a defective fetus. The medical steward presents the facts to the parents and counsels them regarding the consequences of allowing the fetus to go to term and makes recommendations for alternative courses of action.[15] If the decision is made to continue the pregnancy, then it is highly possible that nature will abort the defective fetus. When spontaneous abortion is likely, the wisdom of valiant efforts to carry the fetus to term must be questioned and the parents so advised. If a defective fetus is carried to term, heroic efforts may be required to keep it alive, with great cost in effort and money. Is it good stewardship to keep such a fetus alive at such great cost? And what will be the eventual quality of life for the growing child? Will a decision have to be made as to whether life-support systems should be withdrawn from a defective newborn? Each case must be examined on its own merits, with all due consideration for the rights of the parents, the rights of society, and the quality of life of the child-to-be.

It is evident that nature makes mistakes, as in the obvious case of lethal genetic disease and gross birth defects. Thus, some newborns have abnormalities that are incompatible with life, while others may require much support with a very questionable quality of life ahead. Great responsibility is called for in planning the managment of the fetus or newborn found to be seriously impaired. The preservation of mere vegetative life is no more indicated here than it is at the other end of life, and the medical steward must be prepared to work in this area, utilizing the associated roles of counselor and comforter.

There is an element of pathos to the entire subject of abortion which most physicians share. I know of no one who likes abortion as such, and I have never heard anyone talk about a "good" abortion or express pride over having performed one. Abortion is a procedure of last resort and an admission of the failure of other controls. Yet, in some overpopulated countries, even for the purpose of population control, it is the only effective remedy available. Abortion may be the only course open to women in some cultures where contraception is not favored by males. Certainly this is an area in which medical stewards can work for reform by public education, family planning, and improved pre-natal care. At the same time, the medical steward will not shrink from recommending medically indicated abortions or euthanasia for the newborn. Actions such as these are as much an act of loving concern as the relief of pain or removal of a diseased organ.[16]

To exercise any effective controls over the gene pool, repro-duction, and other troublesome areas which contribute to the genetic disease problem, we must contend with a Western cul-tural neurosis or obsession, especially in this country, which emphasizes individual rights to the point of minimizing group rights or the rights of society. Unhappily, we fail to stress the importance of individual responsibility which goes hand-in-hand with rights. In point of fact, we do have group rights also, but they are somehow secondary to those of the individual. For example, we have the law of eminent domain, where private property can be expropriated for the good of the state, and so we know the principle even though it is not a popular one to enforce. Immunization laws and those requiring the isolation of those with communicable diseases are other examples of interest in the collective good, but these too are often unpopular and resisted. Laws to require genetic screening, sterilization, and abortion are going to be difficult to pass and enforce, but what choice have we? Clearly there is a collective good in holding down genetic disease, and there is danger for posterity if we don't.

Insofar as the legality of abortion and euthanasia of the defective newborn is concerned, the courts have held that a fetus has no rights until it reaches the point of viability, defined as the age at which it may sustain an independent existence outside the mother. Once born, the child assumes some rights but not the full panoply of rights accorded an adult. For example, some jurisdictions have allowed passive euthanasia of the newborn, meaning that all life support could be withdrawn in some instances, with the consent of the parents. This right of consent of the parents to euthanasia of a child is not absolute but only holds in situations where the infant has zero or little chance for any quality of life. In cases where parents want to withhold life-saving procedures in the case of a normal child with an acute, life-threatening medical problem, the courts have ruled that treatment must be given. A common example of the foregoing is the case of a child who needs a blood transfusion but whose parents belong to the Jehovah's Witnesses and to whom blood transfusion constitutes sin. Clearly, there is growing judicial support for the quality of life principle.[17]

An interesting development bearing on the responsibility of society and the medical profession for genetic control is the legal concept of wrongful life. This concept holds that it is wrong for society to permit the conception or at least the birth of a child with a serious genetic disease when there was a strong likelihood that this could have been prevented. Several lawsuits have been filed for damages against physicians or other health-care personnel by the parents of defective children who claimed that their genetically transmittable disease traits were known to their physicians, who then failed to advise them against the risk. In other cases physicians failed to advise amniocentesis when there was a strong possibility of a genetically defective fetus. Regardless of the outcomes of specific cases, there seems little doubt that the concept of wrongful life will make us rethink some of our control measures.[18]

What can physicians do? The wrongful life concept appears to be spreading, and there will probably soon be *consumer* pressure for legal controls. Certainly there is going to be increased awareness of this entire genetic issue as a public-health problem, and one can forsee an increasing demand for the voluntary control methods of screening, contraception, sterilization, and abortion. The demand for genetic counseling will also grow. Legal controls will follow slowly.

Deliberate manipulation of genes in the laboratory to control disease-causing traits (genetic engineering) is possible now to a limited degree but will not be practical for a long time. Whenever it does come, it will most probably require legal enforcement because voluntarism does not work well in this country in matters that are perceived as encroaching on individual rights. Some individual sacrifices must be made in any program of eugenics which is dealing with the collective good. One must sometimes sacrifice a cancerous organ in order to save the individual. The science of eugenics fell into disfavor because of some misapplications in social areas early in this century, but this does not nullify its worth which is now needed to lead us out of the jungle of genetic blight. As stewards of health, we had better get cracking.

Is it possible that we can learn something about the rights of the group from another culture and ideology, such as that of mainland China? The Chinese have periodic neighborhood health meetings which all attend to discuss common health problems. It is emphasized that those individuals who fail to take periodic health checks or immunizations or other preventive measures are harming the group. Couples who have more than three children in this overpopulated country are considered harmful to the collective good.[19] In a positive sense the Chinese by dint of mass effort have wiped out the scourge of schistosomiasis and virtually eliminated venereal disease. The fact that the

Chinese have a political ideology which differs from ours should not blind us to the merit of their achievements in health care. These are considerable and could well be imitated. The fact that more than one quarter million children with genetic defects are born in this country each year should concern us as a nation and individually. The probability that these numbers will increase without or collective intervention ought to startle us into positive group action. Can we face this and other issues demanding medical stewardship?

Some critics may contend that there is a wide gulf between the roles of the physician as comforter or advocate and as a steward of health. A shepherd has concern for his flock as well as for the individual sheep. Our earth is a closed ecosystem demanding sound stewardship for all as well as a one-to-one role of comforter and advocate. Since some individuals and groups need more help at times than others, we must use prudence in the allocation and use of scarce resources in or out of the health-care field. Furthermore, there is a balance of individual and group rights which we can achieve if we work at it. We have learned to live this far with the threat of nuclear extinction because it is evident that everyone must work for a sane solution or perish. Meanwhile, we all enjoy the benefits of nuclear energy for peaceful purposes. It is a matter of us all being responsible stewards—can we afford not to be?

CHAPTER 8

THE ETHICS OF HEALTH-CARE PROVISION: RESPONSIBLE MEDICAL STEWARDSHIP

Several years ago, while attending a service club luncheon, I was engaged in conversation with the man on my left, a person I had just met. "What do you do?" was his opening gambit. I told him, and braced myself for the usual retorts, but no. He came back with "Do you know Doc Jones?" I allowed I didn't, I merely recognized that he was one of the local practitioners. "Well, he's a damned good doctor," continued my friend. Intrigued by his testimonial, it was my turn to ask: "Where'd he go to medical school?" "Beats me," he said, "but he's a good doctor." Feeling a mild irritation by now, I asked, "Well, where did he take his internship?" He didn't know. "Any specialty training?" Again, he didn't know. Fully exasperated by now, I finally asked, "Well, then, how do you know he's a good doctor?" His answer: "Any time I ask him, he makes a house call."

This man's assessment of what made his doctor good is a partial answer to what constitutes the ethics of health-care provision. His physician's care was judged by his caring, judged in this case by his willingness to make house calls. This is not an isolated case; many a successful imposter or quack is considered a good doctor by his patients because of his perceived willingness to serve. Similarly, it has been noted that physicians who communicate well are perceived by patients as being more humanitarian. So, the old adage that health care begins with caring for the patient might be revised to read: "Health care begins with not only caring for the patient but appearing to care." Caring is an important part of quality health care.[1]

In the history of health care in this country, at various times American medicine has appeared indifferent to the health needs of the poor; of appearing not to care. Remember how often organized medicine has opposed health-care legislation for the poor and elderly? Whether the medical profession really cared is not the point; in the best therapeutic relationship the physician must appear to care; it is actually a part of that which we call competence. Good will can hardly prevail if the medicial profession does not appear to care. The medical profession has a long tradition of responsibility to both the individual patient and to society, and it is in this light that our current societal responsibilities must be examined.

HEALTH CARE AS A RIGHT

We live today in a time when human rights are constantly quoted or mentioned. The television cop tells his partner after the arrest of a suspect: "Read him his rights." In past years we have had civil rights, rights to minimum wages, rights to decent housing, the right to breathe pure air, patients' rights, and women's rights to mention but a few, and we are now hearing more and more about rights to health and health care.

There are differing views on the notion of a right to health. Donnie Self argues that health is a moral right of everyone because it is natural, inalienable, and inseparable from existence itself and no one should have it taken away. However, he believes that a right to health *care* is generally only a legal right based on a contract with an individual, an institution, or the government which has previously been made. But Self feels that physicians, by distinction, have a moral obligation to provide health care to those who need it because of their privileged status and professional tradition.[2] Thus, although patients have no right to demand health care from an individual physician, the medical profession corporately has a moral obligation to provide health care to society. I personally agree with these views but there are physicians who strongly disagree. In a forceful statement surgeon Robert Sade declares that no one has a right to health care because this would cause the state to force physicians to provide that care, a situation incompatable with the individual rights of physicians as citizens; rights guaranteed by the Constitution.[3] Sade appears to overlook the obligations imposed by the Hippocratic legacy and the privileged status, if not the professional education, which society confers on a physician.

Daniel Callahan believes that a right to health cannot be guaranteed or provided and therefore the notion is of little use in a practical sense. He reviews the various terms associated with rights in the health care field and concludes, like Self, that most would agree that a right to health care is a reasonable and desirable goal which the state should continue to pursue.[4] Meanwhile, the most realistic and visible goal is for the right of all of equal *access* to health care. Now the problems begin, for, as one wag put it, how much of what is enough for whom and who decides?

It is doubtful that anyone raised in the American tradition would deny any individual the right to seek health care, and everyone would agree that there should be enough of it for all, regardless of socioeconomic status. Having established the idea of equal access to health care for all as a right, as the old story goes, we must now haggle over the price.

Organized medicine fears that the price may be the loss of professional independence and the intrusion of the federal and state governments into the sacrosanct patient-physician relationship—with an accompanying loss of confidentiality, loss of income, bureaucratic meddling, and inability of the patient to chose his own physician. The conservatives and antiwelfare group view the price as too high, saying the costs will be excessive, and future generations will be unable to pay for whatever socialized programs are instituted. They point to the current and projected deficits of present Social Security programs, including Medicare and Medicaid. For the liberals the price is right because of the failure of the free market system of medicine to adequately provide equal care to all, and they push for reforms that are often hastily conceived and poorly executed. There are, of course, valid reasons for all of these fears, which only brings home forcibly the fact that careful planning, implementation and monitoring are necessary if we are to avoid these excesses.

With the above in mind, let's look at the status of health care in this country with regard to inequalities, supply, economic and geographic factors, patterns of utilization, and health man-power.

BARRIERS TO HEALTH CARE

Insofar as utilization of health-care facilities is concerned, three factors must be considered: are they available, accessible, and acceptable? If a facility is available, it exists somewhere. If it is accessible it may be reached by one who needs health care within a reasonable length of time. Acceptability indicates the level of satisfaction felt by the patients with the services they receive. Some additional factors under acceptability include economic, racial, eligibility, and perception of need.

The economic factor simply means that the patient either can afford to pay for the care or cannot. Studies have shown that minority group members feel stigmatized and inferior to some degree and this makes some of them hesitate to use a given medical facility, even if eligible for care there. For some years it was erroneously assumed that minority groups wanted to attend medical facilities staffed by their own ethnic group, but at least one study has refuted this and, indeed, some minorities view such an assumption as discriminatory.[5] One new hospital was built primarily for use by blacks, but after the civil rights struggle of the 1960s, this facility was viewed as discriminatory, and it finally had to close. If the patient can't afford medical care at a given facility, is he eligible for care at a reduced cost or no cost?

What must he do to establish eligibility? Are there long lines and waits? How is he treated? Is the interview demeaning? Patients tend to shun facilities that treat them poorly.

One of the major barriers to health care utilization is ignorance of many of the several health services which are available and why they should be visited. Removal of this barrier will require an adequate and aggressive program of health education especially for the poor, who have the greatest need. For example, they need to know about medical facilities and special screening clinics for diseases with a high incidence among them such as diabetes, high blood pressure, obesity, and tuberculosis. They also need to learn the fundamentals and advantages of a healthful lifestyle and about preventive services such as Pap smears, chest films, routine checkups for pregnant women, infants, and young children, and immunizations. Information must be given about warning signs and symptoms which should be investigated such as pain, difficult breathing, fatigue, gain or loss of weight, unusual discharge, or any deviation from feeling well. While it is clear to many of us that such signs and symptoms should be checked at a medical facility, it is a fact of life that many, especially the poor, will fail to do so. Lack of knowledge, a sense of fatalism, and a pattern of life largely unaccustomed to medical care are major reasons for poor utilization of medical services now available to them at low or no cost. Here is a pressing challenge for the ethical tradition of service.

HEALTH MANPOWER PROBLEMS

There is a shortage of physicians in this country which is compounded by a maldistribution both in geographical location and choice of specialty. Until recently there was a decline in the number of new physicians entering primary care fields such as family or general practice, pediatrics, and internal medicine and a crowding in the medical and surgical specialties. Under the free market system there has been a concentration of physicians in the high-income areas and those areas which offer pleasant living conditions. This physician shortage has been a special problem in providing health care to the poor, for too few doctors have been motivated to move into poverty areas or to participate in health-care programs designed to help in these areas. Even though many younger physicians seem more attuned to social issues and seem concerned about correcting social problems and aiding the poor, only a small percentage indicated a willingness to serve in salaried health-care positions in Appalachia or elsewhere.[6] These programs have had chronic problems related to recruiting and keeping well-qualified physicians. Many different incentives have been suggested and tried to relieve this shortage in rural and other underserved regions, but only a few programs have met with even limited success.[7] Two of the most widely used programs have been a monetary incentive and placement of trainees in underserved areas, but the literature does not support either of these as being effective.

For example, plans offering medical students loans without interest or even outright cancellation of debts to those who ultimately locate in underserved areas have not been successful. Generous salaries and fringe benefits and free office space or housing have also proved ineffective. The provision of a training experience in underserved areas for medical trainees has had limited success but deserves further trial. Students who come from rural backgrounds are more apt to locate in rural practices, but this has not been a significant factor in the selection of applicants for medical school. It might be inductively reasoned that if a student from a rural background is selected for an attractive rural training program, he might be more apt to practice in a rural location. On the other hand, recruiting larger numbers of poor and minority students has not been an effective measure against maldistribution since too few of them locate in poor or minority areas.

Furthermore, incentives such as group practice opportunities in rural settings have been both effective and attractive but have been underutilized. In short, there has been too little utilization of incentives shown to be effective coupled with a stubborn resistance to abandon methods which are ineffective. Abraham Flexner stated in 1912 that increasing the number of medical graduates alone would not improve this problem, and although the number of graduating physicians has doubled since World

War II and continues to climb, this has not resulted in any significant improvement in the maldistribution problem. Despite this fact and other evidence, a spokesman for the AMA insists that the private sector of medicine can solve the problem within the free market system.[8] Federal and state governments have poured millions of dollars into programs designed to help solve this problem with questionable cost effectiveness. Why don't we try to attract service-oriented applicants into medicine and work at fortifying that service orientation throughout their training? Service orientation is a vital characteristic of the professional person.

Physician extenders have been used and are proposed to be used for providing more health care in underserved areas. These are nonphysicians, nurses, or others who have had varied amounts of training in the essentials of medical practice and who work under the supervision of a licensed physician who bears the ultimate responsibility for the extender. Such extenders have been used successfully in remote areas, maintaining contact with the supervising physician by telephone or radio. This seems an acceptable solution in some cases, since there are areas which need medical care but in which a physician would rarely, if ever, locate.

The crucial issue in the use of such "mid-level" practitioners is how ethical and how responsible is the supervising physician? There have been too many cases where the extender could not locate the physician or perhaps did not try very hard and other cases where the physician gave the extender virtually total freedom to do as he or she wished. The extender concept is subject to abuse and exploitation and can be no better than the supervising physician. Alleged abuses of this kind have led, sometimes unfortunately, to sharp curtailment of what the extender may legally do. Since the ultimate responsibility for the extender's actions lies with the supervising physician, it is apparent that the medical profession should agree on what the extender may do and monitor itself on the ethical use of all extenders.

One answer to the health manpower problem in our hospitals and underserved areas has been to permit increasing numbers of foreign medical graduates (FMG) to come into this country.

Many of them initially come to the U.S. for the avowed purpose of graduate training but did not return home afterward and entered practice here. For several years the FMG tended to specialize rather than enter primary care and gravitated toward urban areas. In response to the need for more physicians, the federal government relaxed its immigration and visa requirements for the FMG, and an increasing tide of them entered this country in the decade prior to 1976; there were 31,000 here in 1963 and 68,000 in 1972. In 1975 about 20 percent of all physicians in the United States were FMGs and had the trend continued, it would be closer to 50 percent now.[9] Many FMGs were exploited by hospitals and other institutions of questionable quality, which only required, to use Derbyshire's phrase, some "warm bodies in white coats." Derbyshire was one of the few authorities who protested the exploitation of the FMG and advocated firm measures for improving the quality of those permitted to work here.[10]

The FMG, generally speaking, has not had the quality of training provided in the American system. Furthermore, the FMG often lacks fluency in English and a knowledge of our customs and culture. Ability to communicate well is an important part of competence and many FMG lack that ability. Furthermore, they are viewed as "foreigners" by some segments of our population which often reduces their effectiveness. However, in all fairness to the FMGs, their intellectual abilities have been impressive. Furthermore, there is now evidence that the FMGs are more evenly distributed relative to the population, at least in Maryland, than the United States medical graduates.[11] Two other studies have compared the professional performance of United States medical gradutes and FMGs as (1) attending physicians and (2) as house staff physicians; no significant differences were noted between the two groups.[12] On balance, it does not appear that the FMG offers a satisfactory long range solution to the health manpower problem.

Some of this discussion is now academic, since the Health Manpower Act of 1976 has stated that FMGs are no longer "desirable aliens," as it is projected that commencing in 1980 there will be sufficient American graduates to supply our needs.[13] This sharp reduction of the FMG influx has caused a predictable reaction from hospitals which still face deficits in their house staffs, but many of these institutions were the former exploiters of the FMG. There is now no serious manpower shortage and because of the FMG restriction the overall quality of care should be improved. However, in 1981 there is still a maldistribution problem.

There is another important ethical issue in the FMG "solution." Until 1976 this country actively solicited the immigration of FMGs who often came from countries which had a much more serious health manpower crisis than the U.S. Paradoxically, we often sent teams of physicians and other health-care personnel to these same countries to help relieve their manpower problems! We sent a continuous stream of medical volunteers to South Viet Nam during the war because of their appalling shortage of native physicians but finally permitted some 350 of their physicians, about one-fifth of their total number, to enter this country in 1975 as "political refugees." The AMA has openly supported the immigration of these so-called refugees, probably in response to the wishes of its membership who wanted more FMGs as hospital house officers.[14] This policy was terrible international public relations at best and harmful to both countries.

There has also been a shortage of physicians in primary care, meaning general physicians who are the first point of contact the patient makes with the medical establishment. In an effort to relieve this shortage and/or maldistribution, the government has given liberal financial support to a number of family practice training programs, which have burgeoned in this country in the past decade. The training or residency requirement for this "unspecialized specialty" is three years in a qualified program. There have been problems with this solution right from the start. In order for the programs to prove their academic worth within a medical center, the founders set up stringent guidelines for the training requirements and then recruited academically oriented physicians to manage the programs. Furthermore, only first-rate academic trainees were accepted. In their preoccupation with establishing academic excellence, many programs lost sight of their goal to train physicians for primary care of families. Furthermore, most of these programs are attached to medical centers usually located in large urban areas where the emphasis is on tertiary or super-specialized medical care; an environment which does not approximate the small-town or rural communities where physicians are badly needed.[15]

It is little wonder that this approach has not succeeded in placing many physicians in underserved areas. Physicians tend to practice in the same size city in which they train. After a trainee has worked in a medical center environment for three years and grown accustomed to all the sophisticated gadgetry plus the luxury of a wealth of specialists within easy calling range, he is not going out to Haystack, U.S.A.* on his own, or any other area which lacks the practice amenities and life-style to which he has grown accustomed. Furthermore, he is rarely challenged anywhere in his training by the joys of serving where he is badly needed. Although the guidelines for family practice programs call for an adequate exposure to the social and community aspects of medical practice, too few trainees, in fact, ever get an experience in an underserved area. A rural experience in their training is not required, despite the fact that these programs all receive public funding, at least in part, to relieve the rural physician shortage. Small wonder that advertisements like the following are appearing (1976):

Family Practice: Age 28, married, completing family practice residency.** Will be board eligible 1977. Licensed in S.C. Seeks partnership, solo, or single-specialty group in large metropolitan area. Minimum first-year income, $50,000.

South Carolina and New Mexico are relatively poor states with a large rural population and a marked shortage of physicians. Both have family practice programs at their state medical centers. As a medical administrator who has worked in both states, I found it extremely difficult to recruit qualified physicians, nor could I interest either state's family practice program in sending trainees to our clinics. The clinics in both states were of the rural neighborhood-health-center type and provided health care to the medically indigent. The story was the same in both states; the

*A mythical small rural community.
**Some slight editing in the text was performed to protect the guilty.

programs were not interested in our problems, and they did not want to use us in a teaching capacity. The residents I interviewed did not seem particularly interested in the teaching opportunities we offered, nor could I recruit them as staff physicians when they finished their training. In talking to the undergraduates I found that most of them were unaware that our clinics provided a practice experience which they could choose if they wished. If my experience in these two states is typical, and I have no reason to think it is not, then these publically-funded programs are failing to provide the relief that was intended. In 1981, there remain areas that need physicians and still cannot attract them.

There are other studies that cast doubt on the ability of family medicine training programs alone to produce more family practitioners.[16] They suggest that a restructuring of emphasis and attitude in medical education is necessary if these programs are to accomplish their goal. Another study casts doubt on the ability of other primary care (pediatrics, internal medicine, obstetrics) training programs to hold former trainees in primary care once they enter private practice. A considerable number of these former trainees had changed into more restrictive specialties and therefore did less primary care.[17] Federal funds have been given to medical residency training programs where at least 35 percent of the trainees were in primary care programs but the success of this financial incentive is dubious.

The Graduate Medical Education National Advisory Committee (GMENAC) was established by the U.S. Department of Health, Education and Welfare (HEW) in 1976 in part to provide advice to the secretary on the number of physicians needed in this country and in what specialties and locations. Several advisory reports have been issued by GMENAC; the most recent and probably the most controversial was released in late 1980.* This report to the secretary, of what is now called the Department of Health and Human Services, predicts a surplus of 70,000 physicians by 1990. The surplus will be in fifteen specialties, mostly surgical, with a shortage in four, and a near balance in eight. To

---

*Report of the Graduate Medical Education National Advisory Committee to the Secretary, Department of Health and Human Services, Vol. 1, GMENAC Summary Report. Washington, D. C.: U. S. Government Printing Office, (September 1980).

correct these predicted manpower problems GMENAC made several recommendations, including banning most new, foreign medical graduates (whether or not U.S. citizens) from entering practice in this country. It was also recommended that medical school enrollment be held at its present level with an ultimate reduction of 3,000 students by 1984. It was further recommended that the medical education community find some means to encourage medical students and graduate physicians to enter one of the specialities where shortages are predicted or to enter a primary care specialty. In addition, those medical students still in training should be advised of the current needs as they exist within the various specialties and in what geographical locations around the country. Federal funding should be reduced to medical education in accordance with these recommendations. It is too early to tell how accurate GMENAC's predictions are or what the results of their recommendations may be, but while the medical education community agrees with many of these recommendations it clearly feels threatened.** Obviously, there will be problems if these predictions are valid, including a rise in health-care costs, if corrective measures are not taken. This will involve some sacrifice in accordance with sound stewardship principles.

SOME OTHER INEQUALITIES IN HEALTH CARE

Until relatively recently the free market system of medical care predominated in this country, which largely meant that those who could afford it received good medical care while those who could not afford it got little or none and much of what they did get was of questionable quality. In between were those of average means who could not afford the health care needed for extensive or catastrophic illness. Furthermore, most of our more affluent citizens have health care insurance while two-thirds of the poor do not; those who need it the most have it the least.

There are many places in our country, urban and rural, where health-care facilities and personnel are minimal or absent or access may be difficult because of long distances, lack of trans-

**Editorial, "Response to the GMENAC Report," *Journal of Medical Education* 56 (April 1981): 368-71.

portation, or other problems. Many people reared in poverty see
a physician only as a last resort, with chronic disorders and
painful afflictions accepted as a way of life. Rural or urban poverty areas have rates of alcoholism, mental disease, chronic disease, and infant mortality roughly twice that of areas where
middle- and upper-income classes prevail. Proponents of free
market medicine should spend some time in these poverty areas
and note for themselves the impact of poverty on health. Many
of these medically underserved poverty areas produce much of
the nation's wealth. The coal producing areas of Appalachia
provide a case in point; judging by the wealth which comes out of
the ground, there should be excellent health care for all. Sadly,
the health statistics do not agree.

There is a further irony in the case of Appalachia. Although
the United Mine Workers started what was one of the model
comprehensive health-care plans for its members in the 1950s,
the plan was sharply curtailed within a few years, and the
reduced benefits were a major issue in the crippling UMW strike
of 1977-78. These health-care plans became bankrupt because of
financial juggling of their funds by union officials and some
machinations by the coal industry.[18]

Migrant workers are another low-income group which produces much of this country's agricultural wealth, but their health
statistics are as abysmal as those of the miners: little of the
wealth they produce is ever returned to them in terms of decent
health care.[19]

Such conditions exist largely because of the habitual exploitation of these workers who have little control over the limited
health-care facilities available: management and landowners are
commonly overrepresented on the managing boards of these
facilities while the workers have little or token representation.[20]

The health statistics for the urban poor are not much better.
The well-known urban blight with resultant flight of the more
affluent to the suburbs has taken the best medical-care facilities
and professionals along, leaving the ghetto areas markedly
underserved. The resultant maldistribution of health-care professionals and facilities has created a problem for the poor,
whether urban or rural.

Our elderly people form another group whose health-care needs are poorly provided. These people, many of whom are in retirement situations, live on fixed incomes or pensions which are being steadily eroded by inflation. Many in this group have chronic diseases which often require expensive hospital or nursing-home care which serves to compound their problems.

SOME ATTEMPTED SOLUTIONS

The United States Congress has been increasingly aware of the plight of migrant workers and has been voting ever-larger appropriations to provide health care and other services for them. Some of the workers residing in Florida have been provided special coverage by one of the Blue Cross-Blue Shield programs; such coverage is good wherever the worker migrates. Various health-care facilities in several states have been authorized to provide services to eligible workers. In the southwest a network of clinics has been established solely for the use of migrant workers. The East Coast Migrant Health Project in Washington, D.C. is assisting health-care facilities in several states to provide more care. Practically all of these programs have short-term funding from the Department of HEW, but there are other voluntary agencies, some of which provide care without federal support. However, the bulk of these programs are new, limited in scope, and do not emphasize preventive medicine or patient education; the approach is still basically one of episodic care. Furthermore, future funding for these programs is uncertain, and there is no uniform approach to present and future needs of these workers. Their mobility during the crop seasons presents a real problem, and the challenge is to provide more comprehensive care including prevention and the teaching of good basic health habits. Several volunteer medical groups provide help but the challenge is still far from met.

In the past two decades a number of federally subsidized clinics have sprung up in underserved rural and urban areas. Known as community health centers or neighborhood health centers, they are designed to provide care to the poor and those on marginal incomes. In some areas they provide care for the migrant workers. These centers are funded on the basis of annual grants by the Department of Health and Human Services) (formerly HEW). The original intent was that these centers would generate enough income, once established, to be self-sustaining, but this hope has not been realized. Clinic fees are charged according to one's income, and some of these charges are paid by third party carriers, private insurance, and other federal agencies such as Medicaid. These centers are governed by boards consisting of community residents, and staff personnel are recruited from the area as much as possible.

Although these neighborhood health centers were designed to provide comprehensive care (dentistry, medicine, nursing, sanitation and environmental services, social services, home health services, patient education, and others), this may vary greatly from one center to another, and the costs per patient visit have remained high. There have been many problems with recruiting and keeping competent staffs, especially physicians and nurses, and personnel problems have generally plagued these clinics. There is often considerable tension between the physicians and lay administrators; the latter are often seen by the physicians as not knowledgeable and uncaring about the needs and problems of the medical staff. The future of these centers is unclear since their poor cost-effectiveness and personnel problems have made them the targets of critics, especially from organized medicine and Congress. Having worked with these centers for several years, I am reasonably familiar with them and have misgivings about their degree of success. There is no question of the need, and they have provided health care of variable quality in areas that previously had little or none. However, it must be said that there have been excesses, such as job patronage for minority members of the community, some of whom are incompetent but are still retained, and there have been questionable handling and disbursing of funds. If these centers could be made more efficient all around, they would offer a reasonable model for health-care delivery.[21]

LESSONS FROM MEDICARE AND MEDICAID

In view of the evidence that marked inequality of health care does exist in this country and the "rights" atmosphere of the

1960s, the climate was favorable for the passage of the Medicare-Medicaid (Title XVIII and XIX of the Social Security Act) legislation in 1965. These laws represented an attempt by Congress to correct a social injustice in the area of health care in the same spirit that legislation was being enacted to insure civil rights, minimum wages, and better housing. At last the poor and the elderly would have the health care they needed. In the enthusiasm attending the passage of Medicare-Medicaid, few could predict the mess that lay ahead, especially for the Medicaid program.

In essence, the Medicare acts provided medical care, with certain limitations and exclusions, for those who had retired under the Social Security system. The Medicare benefits were uniform from one state to another: the program was fully funded by the Social Security Administration, and control was retained by the federal government. Medicaid, by distinction, was an optional program for each state designed to provide medical-care benefits for those poor who were receiving public assistance from the state. Funding was jointly provided by the state and federal governments, but control, including eligibility requirements and benefits, was largely left to each participating state. Benefits thus vary from state to state, and only one state, Arizona, is not participating in the program. It should be noted that some states have had funding problems and have literally run out of money from time to time.

There was a good deal of confusion in the early days of these programs, and while eligibility rules were being established for Medicaid, there was underutilization of these services by the poor. There was also the stigma of "welfare" attached to these new programs, and many eligible recipients continued to go the the older, free clinic facilities or somehow paid for their own care. Once the programs got underway, however, this utilization rate began to rise as the onus of "welfare medicine" began to disappear, and more people found out they were eligible.

Medicaid would pay for services provided by a private practitioner in his own office, and this did much to increase the acceptability of the program to the patient. Utilization rates by the poor now equal or exceed those by the more affluent, who provide their own health care. Considering the poorer health of those served by Medicaid, these utilization figures are still too low in

terms of what many of them require for their conditions, but
certainly these increased utilization figures are encouraging.[22] In
addition, the health statistics of the poor have begun to improve.[23]
For example, infant mortality was down 33 percent from 1965 to
1974, with an even better reduction of the death rate in the first
year of life, a period in which high rates have historically been
associated with families of the poor. There was a 14 percent
decrease in the death rate of young children between 1965 and
1973, while age-adjusted death rates for the entire population
were down 10 percent between 1964 and 1974. While many
factors have undoubtedly contributed to these improved figures,
it is at least plausible to attribute some of this to the improved
utilization of health-care services provided by Medicare and
Medicaid.

But the costs soon began to mount way above the projection.
Why? For one thing, the total number of recipients increased. In
the ten-year period since Medicare-Medicaid was begun, inflation also has had an effect. Hospital and other custodial health-
care institutional costs rose, 155 percent between 1960 and 1970,
while the cost of living rose some 31 percent. Hospital and
nursing home costs were responsible for the bulk of the increase.
Hospital costs in particular have risen greatly for many reasons:
there has been a rush for increasingly expensive laboratory and
other medical equipment and practically every hospital has
insisted on obtaining the latest equipment, which often results in
neighboring hospitals having the same sophisticated, costly, and
seldom-used equipment.

There was a time when hospital employees were among the
lowest paid group you could find; much of the work was even
done by volunteers. Times have changed; the salaries of nursing
and auxilliary staffs have risen, and a growing number of well-
paid administrators and technicians have been added to the hospital payroll. As the costs rose, the hospitals raised the room rates
and the third party carriers, (the insurance companies and other
responsible parties) paid the new rates—and passed the increased
cost along to the consumer in the form of higher premiums or
taxes. Physicians who admitted patients to hospitals demanded
more and more of the equipment and technology which seemed

fashionable with no regard for the costs. In many cases they overutilized the hospitals by keeping patients too long, by admitting patients who could have been treated in an office setting or a nursing home, and by ordering expensive and often unnecessary tests, all of which contributed to the well-known inflationary spiral.

In other sectors of the new socialized programs, the cost statistics were similar. Between 1966 and 1973, the average medical costs per year of those over 65 rose from $45 to $1,044, with Medicare paying between 32 percent and 46 percent of these costs. The administrative chores for Medicare-Medicaid, the processing and checking of claims, monitoring of utilization, establishment of "reasonable" reinbursement, and other paper work are handled by the so-called "intermediaries"; Blue Cross, Blue Shield, private insurance companies, and other private corporations. The cost of these service by intermediaries for Medicare alone was some $350 million in 1976. One congressional investigation after another has been critical of these intermediaries, finding generally that they have been too lax in curbing overutilization and permissive in allowing physicians and hospitals to overcharge.

Another factor contributing to rising costs has been widespread fraud and abuse by some medical providers; medical doctors, chiropractors, and osteopathic physicians. Some of healthcare institutions, especially nursing homes, have been equally guilty. This problem has existed since Medicare-Medicaid began but has gotten worse and takes many forms. Physicians may bill for more than they actually provide, or they may charge for services never performed. More pernicious is the Medicaid "mill", where a high volume of patients is rammed through a medical office, where they receive many questionable injections, laboratory examinations, X rays, and procedures of various kinds. Senator Frank Moss personally conducted an investigation of these mills in 1977 and was himself the victim of several unnecessary procedures.[24] Some of the laboratories investigated turned out to be converted garages with the most meager and primitive equipment. Rebates to medical providers and nursing homes from medical suppliers, laboratories, and pharmacies were commonplace. One chiropractor, convicted for fraud in the running of several Medicaid mills, told a Senate committee that the Medicaid program itself was to blame, citing the fee-for-service system as placing temptation right in the provider's path. A common rationalization for this fraud and abuse is that since Medicaid pays lower than usual and customary fees, one must resort to such unethical practices, but the fact is that the effects of such actions on the health of the patients is ignored.

The Medicaid mills and other abuses of the Medicaid program were the subject of a special television report in 1976 which presented bountiful evidence of these abuses. In this presentation the president of the AMA was interviewed and blandly declared that only a few physicians were involved.[25] A few? Shortly afterward, in the article cited above, Senator Moss estimated that the fraud in Medicaid amounted to 10 percent, or 1.7 billion dollars a year! Evidence of fraud and abuse of the social medicine programs continues to mount, but little more has been done to curb it. A more recent study, which was supported by federal funds, found that most large Medicaid practices did not appear to be Medicaid mills. However, the study did find that a "credentials gap" existed in that the medical providers were dominated by less qualified physicians and that physicians with large Medicaid practices tended to be older, non-board certified, and graduates of foreign medical schools.[26]

A common diversionary tactic by critics and those who abuse these programs has been to claim that it is the recipients or patients who abuse the programs and run the costs up by over-utilizing the services and coming to the physician for the most minor complaint. Such frivolous use or overuse by recipients has been miniscule, according to the real authorities.[27] The main reason for the rising costs, inflation and numbers of eligibles aside, has been provider abuse and especially overutilization of hospitals and nursing homes by health-care providers. Such institutional care continues to account for the biggest chunk of the health-care dollar

Another factor in the rising costs of social medical programs has been the increasing number of people in the over 65 population; some 22 million in 1976, which is twice the number in 1966.

Medicaid estimates that three out of five dollars go for services to aged or disabled adults, while 35 percent of all payments go for services provided in skilled and intermediate nursing-care facilities. This trend is projected to continue for the next forty to fifty years, which means the costs will become more critical as times passes. There are already proposals for taxing Social Security payments and for extending the retirement age to 68. Clearly these Social Security programs are facing a serious problem of funding.

INSTITUTIONAL CARE PROBLEMS

We have alluded several times to the disproportionate costs for hospital and nursing home care, especially in the social medicine programs. Many old people are in institutions of various kinds because society does not want them at home. Physicians, as members of society, naturally reflect some of this attitude toward the aged or chronically ill. Patients covered under the Medicare-Medicaid programs must be certified by a physician that institutional care is needed for health reasons and then periodically recertified. In actuality many of these patients do not need expensive nursing-home or hospital care but are often there because of an inadvertent conspiracy. The next-of-kin and physicians find it easy to put the old and "unfit" away, and there are plenty of institutions eager to receive them; a hospital or nursing-home administrator's nightmare is one of empty beds.

There are several different levels of health care, beginning with the most expensive, the hospital. Many hospitalized patients can be cared for in nursing homes, and many nursing-home patients could be discharged to the care of certified nursing homes, or given home health services, or simply discharged from all care because they are well. Home-health services provide needed care in the home by qualified personnel at greatly reduced cost, and in many cases this is all the care the patient requires. For commercial and attitudinal reasons there is often resistance to change in the level of care.

Patients who are cared for in nursing homes under federally supported Medicaid and Medicare programs must have certification and periodic recertification by a physician for the need of such care. Review or utilization committees such as PSRO's check on each patient to see that such care is needed and actually provided. All such committees have physician members or consultants. If the committee decides that a change or discharge is needed, the family and physician of the patient are notified and may challenge the intended change. However desirable such review may be it will not lessen the need for a change of attitude on the part of society, the medical profession, and the institutional health care industry.

For many reasons the actual care provided in some nursing homes is shockingly bad. The nursing home industry in this country has been lucrative for many operators and a nightmare for many of the residents. The scandals which have been so prevalent in the nursing home industry have been well-documented.[28] It is evident that it is the health-care providers, especially the physicians, who must be the leaders in bringing about reform. It is the physician who must admit or discharge the patient and who is directly responsible for the utilization of health-care institutions. Physicians, as conservers and stewards, must be economical in the ordering of hospital and nursing home admissions, the use of laboratories, X rays, expensive procedures, and drugs. Furthermore, as a professional who is a transmitter of culture and opinion-maker, the physician is obligated to resist the trend of society to follow the Toilet Assumption and make others aware of the place and contributions of the elderly in community and family life.

In an effort to improve the quality of care and its soaring costs, the government has required that states participating in Medicare-Medicaid institute a Professional Standards Review Organization (PSRO). Normally comprised of physicians and implemented by state medical societies, the PSRO is a sort of super peer review committee for a given area and maintains a close watch on hospital utilization as well as ambulatory health care. Physicians who wish to participate in social medicine programs must adhere to guidelines and are sometimes called on to justify their patient care management. If justification is not adequate, the claim for payment is rejected.

There have been some cries of outrage from the medical community about the PSROs, so that whereas most of the state medical societies have implemented them, some others have refused. The federal government has replied that if the state medical societies don't staff the PSROs, then they will be staffed by nonphysicians. After some years of experience with PSROs, there is controversy over their value. They have not been effective in reducing costs, but they appear to have reduced some of the abuse by improving the quality of care provided and by reducing unnecessary tests and treatments. Faced with the peer review that the PSRO provides, many physicians will adhere to the guidelines for good medical practice. Meanwhile, some authorities are convinced that the PSRO approach won't work, at least in containing costs.[29]

The terrible irony in the physician abuse of the Medicare-Medicaid programs is that the practice is depriving many of the poor of health services they desperately need. The increase in costs, partly as a result of this abuse, has caused some states to curtail benefits or reduce the numbers of those eligible for Medicaid; a right reserved to the states. It is estimated that some 40 million impoverished Americans or those with borderline incomes who are "medically indigent" are not now receiving Medicaid benefits. The medical profession must share the guilt for this tragedy.[30]

If peer review methods won't curb the costs and abuses, what then? It may be necessary to develop another care system for the poor and aged, or, indeed, a new unified health system for the country. However, in the spirit of the Hippocratic legacy, it seems that the medical steward's approach to this complex problem should be to appeal to one another—provider to provider—to follow medicine's ethical tradition and be something and somebody "very special" again. This does not mean to establish an elitist group but rather to regain the professional pride that was known to Hippocrates and represents a fulfillment of *philia*. There is a terrible urgency for this self-healing because of society's growing annoyance with the entire medical enterprise. The warnings abound everywhere, and medicine had best be at the business of setting its house in order.

ETHICS OF COST CONTAINMENT

Any discussion of health-care costs must start with the realization that there is no such thing as a free lunch. There are many good arguments for more health care, but there is no way to expand health care without increasing costs. Inflation seems to always be with us and is not, *per se*, the cause of rising costs. On the other hand, the expanding health-care establishment is one of the leading causes of inflation, especially the hospital sector. However, there are some methods available that could possibly contain health-care costs within reasonable limits.

It appears that peer review, as presently conducted, is not an effective instrument for cost containment, but it is capable of improving the quality of care. Effective peer review requires some education in the basics of medical economics and cost containment on the part of those who sit on the review committees. When committees are knowledgeable, there is some hope for containing costs, and this will succeed to the degree that practicing physicians are also made cost-conscious. The reasons are many for this ignorance, but today one of the reasons is an almost universal fear of malpractice litigation, a fear that makes physicians overutilize hospitals and diagnostic facilities so that no one will judge them negligent. There is growing pressure for teaching doctors and medical students more about medical economics and currently a two-year pilot program is underway to educate practicing physicians about medical costs.[31] If physicians can be made cost-conscious, then they are more likely to contain costs in their own practices, and they will be more effective as peer review members who may judge the overutilization of another physician. Since hospital costs are the largest portion of health-care costs and since physicians are the ones who use hospitals, the conclusion is pretty obvious. It is possible that physicians will fail to contain costs, but both society and the Hippocratic legacy are indicating they should. They had better.

Another way of reducing costs, is to reduce unnecessary surgery. The federal government is encouraging second surgical consultations to make certain that proposed surgery is reasonably necessary, and the movement has spread to many health insurance plans that have been faced with runaway health costs. Another method for cutting costs is the growing use of ambulatory surgery centers, where patients are returned home following surgery and not admitted to the hospital. Various insurance carriers, including the Blue Shield and Blue Cross, have encouraged trial of such facilities, and the movement should grow.

Cost-sharing has been suggested as an effective way to reduce costs by requiring the participant in any given health plan or insurance program to share part of the costs, especially hospitalization. This approach is already in effect with Medicare-Medicaid, and some private insurance companies. Use of this method should require continuing health education so that members will know when they should seek health care. Another variety of cost-sharing has been proposed wherein a physician who orders hospitalization and related procedures which later are judged to be unnecessary, shares the cost of such unnecessary care with the patient, the insurance carrier and the hospital.[32] I like the idea but I don't see it as catching on with the medical profession. This practice would certainly curb the overutilizing physician.

Another model of health care that has proved to contain costs is the Health Maintenance Organization (HMO). This approach offers a package of health-care benefits, including ambulatory and hospital services, to either an individual subscriber or to a group for a fixed, prepaid charge. The health services are provided by a panel of full or parttime salaried health-care professionals working together in a group practice. Those who favor this approach, including federal planners, point to the success of plans like Kaiser-Permanente on the West coast, Hospital Insurance Plan of New York, and the Group Health Association in Washington, D.C. These plans have an excellent record of holding down costs while providing quality health care. Hospital utilization and surgical rates are about half of those in the rest of the country without any evidence of increased risk to the patients. Simply stated, it pays the HMOs to keep their patients well.

In this aura of HMO popularity, federal legislation provided funds for feasibility and planning studies for proposed new HMO programs as well as startup money for the first year or two of operation. The experience has been mixed; whereas the established groups often enrolled low-risk populations such as the employees of a given industry, the newer HMOs lacked experience and many of them took on high-risk members. This, with other rising costs, caused many of them to fold. However, others have succeeded and the federal government seems determined that there shall be further funding for HMOs because of their potential for reducing costs. Meanwhile, there have been complaints from some HMOs that they have been boycotted by private physicians and some Blue Cross Blue Shield plans. Overutilization, fraud, and abuse have been evident here as well. Critics have pointed out that if fee-for-service tends to promote overutilization of services, an HMO could as easily underutilize needed care in an effort to reduce costs, but this point has not been demonstrated. Prepaid systems of this type cared for about 4.6 million people in 1968, and the number is much higher now. Subscribers, in general, are pleased with the services they receive from HMOs, and this model of health care must be considered as a suitable alternative for at least certain selected population groups.[33]

Equally important in any effective health-care program or cost-containment effort is the provision of health-care education for the public; the patient and the potential patient. Since health-care costs depend on utilization of services and since health-care education can reduce utilization, the need for education is obvious. Health-care education has been rightly called the "missing link" in health care because it is so little used and its importance not understood. Many people, especially the poor, lack knowledge in matters like basic hygiene, sanitation, sound nutrition, preventive medicine, early warnings of disease, self-health care, and when, where, and how to use health-care facilities.

Most everyone in the health-care game understands the importance of patient education in learning how to live with and care for a chronic disease such as diabetes or hypertension, once diagnosed. Unfortunately, too few health-care professionals understand the advantages of health education which goes beyond existing disease and encourages people to attend special classes where they may learn about the early symptoms and signs of disease and what they may do to help prevent certain disorders. Ignorance of such matters constitutes a definite barrier to effective health-care utilization. The teaching tradition of medicine is not meant only for one's medical colleagues and students; it also demands participation in public programs of health education. The importance of such education has recently been underscored by the creation of a federal interagency group to study and develop ways to train primary care physicians to be effective health-care educators.[34] Physicians simply have not been as active in this field as they should be.

Patient education has taken a rather ironic twist for many members of the middle and upper classes of our Western culture who have become overly dependent on the whole system of medicine or who suffer from what Illich has termed "the medicalization of life." Great numbers of our society have been so indoctrinated by the health care system to believe they must seek professional help for even the simplest complaints that they remain in a state of neurotic dependency, believing that only medical science can relieve their complaints.[35] This delusion has been supported by books, movies, and the mass media in general, which have all erroneously attributed our current good health and longer life solely to medical science. The facts are that improved sanitation, nutrition, and preventive measures such as vaccines have done as much or more than medical care of itself to improve the quality of life. The greatest increase in average life expectancy occurred long before the advent of the so-called miracle drugs of this century. The ironic twist is that sensitive physicians and other health-care professionals must now somehow reeducate these "medicalized" people so that they may learn to care for many of their complaints and ills as did our pioneer forebears—by themselves. Part of the physician's work is to foster health-care independence in his patients by education, and he should not create a fearful dependency in them because of his own neurotic needs or from incorrect beliefs that medical care is constantly needed. One may hope that educational programs for physicians will help correct this delusion.

Finally, it cannot be overemphasized that every patient and citizen has a prime responsibility in the health-care business that has been poorly met.[36] An important part of health education is advising the public how they may live a healthful life and so contribute to their own well-being. Patients must be advised of ways they may contribute to recovery. Some physicians are using what is known as the contract approach to medical practice wherein the patient is told of his condition and diagnosis and the plan of treatment is outlined. The physician tells the patient that he, the doctor, will do everything within his portion of the care program if the patient will do the same. Emphasis is placed on teamwork between patient and health-care provider and "breach of contract" by either party may well scuttle the chances for a successful outcome. This approach takes the patient out of the formerly passive and largely ineffective role that has been the mode for so long and makes him a dynamic member of the team.

Not only the patient in the above contract model but every citizen has an obligation to follow recommended health habits and observe schedules for periodic check-ups and screening. Recommendations for these could be publicized by the mass media, through schools, and doctors' offices, and other public facilities. Veatch carefully examines the issues associated with that small minority that seems so hell-bent on destruction through seemingly voluntary risks to their health and asks whether such high-risk persons ought to bear the cost of truly voluntary health risks.[37] These issues are sharpened by the knowledge that a very small percentage of people are responsible for most of the hospital costs in this country, and most of them are associated with ruinous life-styles, associated with heavy alcoholic consumption, smoking, and failure to follow professional recommendations for care of illness. Such personal habits and life-styles, suboptimal management of prior illness, social factors, or lack of community health-care resources were factors in 78 percent of the hospital admissions in one study.[38] The illness was deemed preventable in 44 percent and could have been controlled on an ambulatory or nonhospital basis in 31 percent had a standard medical regimen been followed. Since a small segment of the population seems responsible for the bulk of health-care costs, it might be prudent to ferret out these offenders and concentrate on their problems, prescribing a sizable dose of health education. As Knowles has said so well:

Life is meant to be enjoyed, and each one of us in the end is still able in our own country to steer his vessel to his own port of desire. But now the costs of individual irresponsibility in health care have become prohibitive. The choice is individual responsibility or social failure. Responsibility and duty must gain some degree of parity with rights and freedom.[39]

A related factor in reducing costs and overutilization is that of self-health care. A few years ago many consumer groups were actively promulgating self-health care by means of publications and brochures, and by practical demonstrations on how to use instruments like the otoscope, stethoscope, and blood pressure cuff. This movement has not expanded to the degree that one might hope; apparently it is hard to "demedicalize" this country. However, self-health care is a pioneer tradition in this country, and many homes formerly contained home health encyclopedias of one sort or another. There is no good reason why self-health care could not be a part of public education right along with the standard hygiene or health courses.

In reflecting about the ethics of the containment of health care costs and the problem of health care for all, a few comments seem in order. With continued inflation and expansion of health care in this country (as seems inevitable) the costs for this care will continue to rise; but one may hope that they will be justified based on what will be provided. However, there are limits, and with the cost of health care now approximating 10 percent of the gross national product, we are hearing warnings from many authorities that this trend cannot continue. Economist Alain G. Enthove, who authored one of the national health insurance proposals considered by the Carter administration, told the AMA board of trustees: "The status quo is untenable. The costs are now large, rising too fast, with government committed to too much, for government not to do what it must to bring them under control."[40] Even the *laissez-faire* spirit of the Reagan administration cannot afford to ignore this continuing threat to galloping inflation.

Illich is undoubtedly right about the medicalization of America; others have noted this country's singular preoccupation with health care. However analyzed, it seems inescapable that the physician is a prime factor in the control of health care costs. It is he or she who must admit patients to hospitals and nursing homes, and order procedures and medications. It is he or she who abuses and defrauds insurance companies and social medical programs. It is he or she who can agitate and work for substantial health-care education, and finally, he or she who must realize that fee-for-service is more conducive to episodic medical care for disease than educational or preventive efforts and contributes to the problem of abuse.

With proper management, effective and comprehensive health care may be provided for low- and middle-income groups by neighborhood health centers and by health maintenance organizations. The fee-for-service method will probably always appeal to some members of society, especially the wealthy, many of whom cling to the notion that you only get what you pay for individually.

One approach to the provision of health care to all is national health insurance (NHI), where the government supports or underwrites the provision of some type of health-care coverage which is similar to any health-care insurance plan. Currently being considered in Congress and considered most likely to pass now is "catastrophic NHI," which would protect citizens from the often ruinous costs of major protracted illness or disability. The range of benefits may be minimal or comprehensive, just as in private plans. The majority of American physicians favor NHI, but the AMA most probably will only support it if based on fee-for-service, an insistence that will retain the present evils of emphasis on episodic illness, minimal preventive or educational efforts, and the temptation to cheat. Any insurance plan based on fee-for-service will tempt some medical providers to cheat, a well-known fact in the insurance industry. A satisfactory form of NHI would require a retainer or salary for the provision of services. Canada has had NHI based on fee-for-service for several years, but there have been plenty of problems. Donabedian has discussed the main issues in NHI and concluded that provision of comprehensive benefits by NHI will necessitate fundamental changes in the organization of health services.[41]

The subject of totally socialized medical care has been pur-
posely avoided until now because it is the last resort of a society
made desperate by the excesses of the present system. In our
present pluralistic system, the physician is the chief controller of
cost and quality. The experience of Britain's socialized medicine
program is that the vast administrative bureaucracy superim-
posed on the health-care providers is responsible for the excessive costs.

However, no one should suppose that the National Health
Service (NHS) in Great Britain is all bad, as its critics, particularly
in this country, sometimes assert. Many physicians and patients
are well satisfied with the program, but many have agreed that
the costs are excessive and the service slow, especially elective
surgery.[42] It must be remembered that our own Medicare-
Medicaid programs were perilously close to financial collapse
several times, and corrective measures had to be taken. Britain's
prime minister, Margaret Thatcher, and her conservative party
were so alarmed over the current cost of the NHS (some 5.5
percent of the GNP or $21 billion in 1979) that they sponsored a
bill scheduled to pass into law in 1980 that will eliminate an entire
segment of the NHS administration and cut other costs.[43] The
same bill would retain some private beds which the Labor party
wished to eliminate and allow construction of some private hospitals. Many NHS physicians serve both private patients and
those covered by the government plan.

Medical sociologist David Mechanic has devoted considerable
space in his book, *Medical Sociology*, to a thoughtful comparison of
the NHS with our own "system." His conclusions are helpful:

The British National Health Service offers people equal access to
national resources when they are sick regardless of their social position
and economic wealth. . . . But the British Health Service has a long way
to go in meeting its ideals and visions; many problems remain, and the
quality of service falls considerably short of what is possible, given the
state of medical knowledge. . . .

In contrast, medical care in America is available on both a higher and
lower level than is typical of England. The finest medical care in the
world is available to those with economic resources and with adequate
information as to where to seek care. But America's resources are less

accessible to the person of lower socio-economic status who require such care than to his counter-part in Britain. It is apparent that both systems of medical care have something to learn from one another, and that some combination of the advantages of both provides an ideal towards which America and Britain can realistically aspire.[44]

We are moving toward a policy of providing health care for an ever-increasing part of that population which has long been underserved. This is as it should be because every physician has an important responsibility to his patient, his community, his country, and the world itself. It's all tied together. One cannot practice individual medicine in a vacuum, there is an ever-widening circle of responsibility up to and including global health where the ultimate goal is to attain the World Health Organization's definition of health which states: "Health is a state of complete physical, mental, and social well-being and not merely the absence of disease or infirmity." Obviously, the patient under one's immediate care has a priority, but this should not exclude a responsibility to society. At times, the one-to-one patient-doctor relationship has prevented physicians from realizing the larger responsibility; there are simply occasions in which the health of the group must come ahead of the needs of the individual.

Concern for the group or community is not always visible in our society where heavy emphasis has traditionally been placed on individual rights, and this occasionally creates needless tension. An example is the failure of some parents to have their children immunized against the common and severe diseases of childhood. Such refusal fails to take into account the rights of the group; if a certain percentage of individuals in a given population lack immunization then the population group itself will lack so-called "herd immunity." The responsibility of parents in cases like this is often discussed in the neighborhood health-group meetings of the mainland Chinese where the good of the group is of primary importance. There is certainly a middle ground between these two extremes.

Finally, physicians must awake to some of the realities in the health-care field which they have largely ignored. There must be a recognition that a pervasive reformation of the health-care system is inevitable. There have been many social changes in the last few decades, and medicine should prepare for its own social changes that will not be long in coming. The federal government will have a major role in the reformation of health care, which must be accepted, but its power must be restricted by the health-care profession; there are plenty of precedents in this country and abroad to tell us why. A spirit of collaboration between medicine and the government is essential for a satisfactory program, a spirit which is in line with the Hippocratic legacy.

Finally, physicians must seek to change the negative approach that has largely dominated the American health scene, wherein too much effort has gone into things like the senseless extension of death, the institutionalization of the unfit and aged, organ transplant, and sophisticated gadgetry which have all given us little return in terms of quality of life or cost-benefit. What is needed is a positive strategy for the nation to replace the some-times negative and often crisis-oriented approach that has been the norm. Lester Breslow offers a prescription:

What would a positive strategy be? It would aim at promoting health, preventing disease, and extending life through developing healthful life-styles, assuring a healthful environment, and turning medicine toward health maintenance. Note that this strategy calls for three main thrusts: (1) promoting personal habits that are favorable to health; (2) countering environmental health hazards; and (3) reorienting medicine to emphasize prevention of disease and maintenance of health.[45]

Any positive health strategy must also demonstrate that the quality of caring is essential to health care. Without a pervasive mentality of caring among all health-care providers, there can be only a mechanistic approach to health care in which quality will be lacking. Caring, as epitomized in the tradition of service, is a part of total competence, yet this idea seems to have escaped the medical profession at times. Is this the case in our current era? The maldistribution problem is not caring, the cheating on social medicine programs is not caring, exploitation of the patient is not caring, neglect of our old people is not caring, and marketplace medicine can be very uncaring.

The true spirit of caring and responsibility will cause the medi-cal profession to correct some of the inequalities that have been discussed here. Organized medicine could ease the manpower problem by voluntary but regulated service in places of need. Also, state governments could easily require periods of service in underserved areas as a condition for licensure. Another alternative is to follow the method of the Mexican medical schools which require a year of service for new graduates in underserved areas before they receive their final degree. I have talked with several American and Mexican graduates of these schools and they all felt the experience was worthwhile.[46] We could easily adopt self-imposed quotas on the numbers of trainees in the various specialties. Medicine has occasionally had a missionary impulse to provide health care to those in need wherever they were; this is an impulse that should be cultivated for the greater good of mankind and the honor of the profession.

Much of the spirit of this chapter is captured in the following:

The honored ideals of the medical profession imply that the responsibilities of the physician extend not only to the individual, but also to society where these responsibilities deserve his interest and participation in activities which have the purpose of improving both the health and well-being of the individual and the community.

This interesting quotation is one of the AMA's ten Principles of Medical Ethics.[47]

CHAPTER 9

EXPERIMENTATION ON HUMANS AND PATIENTS' RIGHTS

EXPERIMENTATION ON HUMAN SUBJECTS

Intimately related to the ethics of health-care provision is the subject of experimentation on humans. Some primitive ancestor of ours noted that certain sick animals got well after ingesting certain herbs and reasoned that humans should try the same remedies. Thus, pharmacology and the clinical trial were born and have continued to aid and trouble us ever since.

Much of modern medicine is empirical, and was formerly based on trial and error on human beings and more recently by more carefully planned and sophisticated studies on laboratory animals. New drugs or pharmaceutical agents or new methods of treatment are usually tested first on animals but ultimately must be tested on humans if the drug or treatment is intended for human use. The need for research on human subjects, or clinical trial, is self-evident if we are to improve the human condition medically.

In recent years clinical trials of new drugs or procedures have come under increased scrutiny and criticism. Although the particular criticism varies from time to time, the principal issue seems to be one of adequate protection for the human trial subject without abandoning the clinical trial method. For example, is the subject adequately informed of the nature of the trial and the risks of being injured and after this information has been provided, has consent been freely given; that is, has "informed consent" truly been obtained? In the event of injury or death, is there an adequate compensatory mechanism for the subject or the next-of-kin? Have coercive methods, however subtle, been used to gain the consent of the subject? Is he underprivileged or disadvantaged in any way so as to render him more subject to coercion or less likely to fully understand the nature of the trial and its risks? Is the trial necessary; that is, is it likely to produce beneficial, new information without a high risk factor? What is its risk/benefit ratio? Is the trial well designed and conducted by competent professionals so that truly valid information is likely to be gathered? These are some of the questions that need to be asked and answered in any proposed experimental studies on humans.

Heated debate has waged for several years over the issue of "informed consent." There are those who would not inform the subject about the trial, holding that to do so would adversely affect the results, and there are those who would not get the consent of the subject prior to the trial. That this has actually happened has been well-documented; in many cases the subjects were not informed, their consent was not obtained, and there were risks involved. At the other pole are those who maintain that full and complete information must be provided to all subjects.

Since trial subjects are sometimes mental patients or minors, informed consent may not be possible to obtain from them, but it must be obtained from the parents or responsible guardians. Obtaining informed consent is a complex matter, requiring different methods than have generally been employed in the past. For example, all the subjects in one clinical trial were fully informed of the nature and risks involved before consent was obtained. Despite the reasonably high intelligence and affluence of the subjects, after 16 weeks only one-third of them could recall receiving any information. The authors concluded that truly informed consent might require continuous reinforcement by some appropriate methods throughout the trial.[1] In another study, the recall rate was similar. In this case, 95 percent wanted to be informed about the trial but 75 percent said they would have consented without such information![2]

Many human trial subjects have been drawn from disadvantaged groups; the poor or ignorant, prisoners, children, and mental patients have often been used. In some clinical trials, control subjects did not receive needed treatment and suffered as a consequence. In other cases coercive methods have been used such as promises, actual or implied, of better treatment, shorter jail terms, and so forth. Such methods are unfair and may affect the validity of the trial results; for example, the subject may be so eager to participate that he will give the responses or report the symptoms which he feels the investigator wants. Many clinical trials have been both criticized and defended because the subjects came from a disadvantaged group and were caused harm or injury as a result of their participation.[3] There certainly was no effort to obtain informed consent in the case of the infamous "medical" experiments conducted under the Nazi regime of the Third Reich. Many people fear a similar thing could happen again without the protection of informed consent; the Nuremberg Code of 1947 was formulated to help prevent such horrors in the future.

Several agencies of the federal government have insisted on informed consent in any clinical trial that they subsidize or that is submitted to support new drug applications. The American Society for Clinical Pharmacology and Therapeutics is vitally concerned with the entire range of human experimentation, and it fully supports the principle of informed consent but wants legislators to be aware of the many difficulties involved in the interpretation and implementation of this complex issue, lest bad law be hastily passed. The organization also believes that ethical and proper clinical research can be conducted on prisoners, mental patients, and children and is concerned that legislation might be passed which would impede necessary research.[4] The American Academy of Pediatrics has supported the principle of ethical research in children including the newborn and the human fetus as long as everything is done to insure the survival of the subject. The Academy further endorses the principle that the benefits to be derived from research must never be given higher priority than respect for the rights of the individual.[5] Judgment as to these priorities may be very different at times.

Since the participation of children and mental patients require the consent of the parents or guardian, special safeguards seem needed. Some have argued that the parents cannot ethically consent to a voluntary procedure or trial when it involves risk to the child, holding that the child might not wish this done. Parents have been given sums of money for permitting their children to be trial subjects; such a tactic can be abused unless there is adequate protection for the interests of the child, such as a trust fund or similar guarantee that the child will receive any funds paid on his behalf. Courts have held that the child is not the exclusive property of his parents so that a child may not be unduly abused, neglected, or maltreated in any way; for example, it is commonplace for a court to remove a child from a home in which he has been abused and place him in a foster home. Likewise, special protection is indicated for mental patients because many times the institution has permitted them to be used as trial subjects. In addition to informed consent, many would now agree that research on children or mental patients should only be done with all due safeguards and only if the research is liable to produce benefits to their particular health impairment or age group.

It is sometimes desirable to compare the results or data gathered from trial subjects with control subjects who did not receive the experimental drug or treatment. Such control subjects must also be protected, for they may also be subject to harm. For example, control subjects commonly have blood samples drawn for purposes of comparison, or food may be withheld or they may be deprived of sleep. In one case a control group of asthmatic children received dummy or placebo injections during the course of a clinical trial to determine the effectiveness of a hyposensitization program. This procedure was potentially dangerous since it deprived some of the children from receiving relief from their usual medications.[6] In another infamous case, treatment was withheld from a control group of syphillitic patients. The practice of using control subjects is a sound one, but the ethics of caring require that they have the same protection as the experimental subjects.

Fortunately, most hospitals in which human experimentation is conducted have ethics committees which alone may permit or deny a proposed trial and also monitor the progress of a clinical trial once it has been started. Many such committees were formed at the insistence of federal agencies which financially supported such research, and informed consent was an additional condition of such funding. Such safeguards are laudable; the regrettable feature is that an economic motive seemed largely responsible for their implementation. As a further protection, it may be necessary to monitor the function of the ethics committees to make certain they do their job.[7] To be effective, an ethics committee should be allowed to judge the merits of a proposed clinical trial and then, if approved, be able to enforce measures designed to protect the subjects.

What if a human subject suffers pain or permanent harm or even death as a result of his participation? The principle of informed consent does not relieve the investigators from the responsibility to provide compensation in such cases. Obviously, medical treatment must be provided for injured subjects, and monetary awards should be provided in the case of prolonged hospitalization, permanent injury, or death. Such compensation should probably be paid through insurance coverage. Carriers could also exercise some supervision over the conduct of the clinical trial and the qualifications of the investigators. The conclusion cannot be escaped: any trial subject deserves the protection of a just compensatory mechanism.

What is the real purpose of a proposed clinical trial involving human experimentation? If it sincerely seeks to prove the merit, or lack of merit, of a treatment or agent, it must be well-designed and be carefully executed by qualified investigators. The risk/ benefit ratio must be warranted; that is, the anticipated results must justify the degree of risk. Hence, a proposed trial of a highly toxic drug for the relief of headache or other minor pain would not be ethically justified, while a trial involving the use of a highly toxic agent for the treatment of cancer would be more easily justified. If the study is frivolous, or unnecessary, it should not be done, but in the "publish or perish" atmosphere of medical science, many such studies appear to have been done. Studies of this nature contribute little or nothing to the benefit of mankind and may have caused unnecessary harm to the subjects.

Thus, a conflict of interest is built into the concept of the clinical trial in that the investigator may be so concerned with what he is trying to prove or disprove or with his own glorification that he overlooks the principle of protection which is due the subject as a fellow human. There is a tension between the physician acting in the traditional role of advocate or therapist and the physician as a clinical investigator.[8] There is often an ethical problem over the risks and the benefits which may accrue to the individual trial subject by his participation and the benefits which may accrue to society. The rights of the individual must be protected, but the needs of society cannot be ignored.

Guttentag has suggested a model of partnership between the investigator and subject as a method for resolving these tensions.[9] Partnership in this sense means a relationship of mutual trust and empathy between investigator and subject that is actually an amplification of the traditional doctor-patient relationship. Such a partnership is difficult to obtain because it is based on trust and *philia*, but it is a needed goal toward which both parties should strive. Meanwhile, ethics committees with adequate enforcement powers must protect the subjects and see that the investigators are properly qualified. Mankind needs the benefits which human experimentation can produce, and it would be unethical not to conduct needed research. But subjects must be fully protected in the spirit of the *philial* partnership model. The ancient adage that the physician should help, or at least do no harm must be remembered while admitting that harm may be done. Such risk is ethically justified in certain cases so long as there is an assumption of the traditional responsibility of caring for the injured subject with just methods of compensation.[10]

Many medical schools do not touch on this problem within the formal curriculum, but many students see clinical trials being conducted or hear about others. This would be an ideal time to present related ethical issues such as the justification for the trial, informed consent, protection, and compensation for the trial subjects. Certainly these topics could be discussed along with the formal course in pharmacology. Erik Erikson feels that the basis or essence of medical ethics is the Golden Rule.[11] The Golden Rule ethic, fully utilized in *philia*, would certainly protect the patients in their relationship with the physician, either as therapist or investigator. Actually, every physician experiments to some degree when he or she treats another person. If a drug or treatment is prescribed, it is because the therapist thinks it may help the patient. Should one modality not work, then another may be tried. But there is no question in this context that the intent of the physician-therapist is to heal or relieve the patient. Ideally, in the fullest sense of caring-in-love, the physician as experimenter or investigator would also protect the *patient* while carrying out the experiment on the *subject*. Realistically, the physician must be either therapist or investigator, but he must protect both patient and subject.

THE PATIENTS' RIGHTS MOVEMENT

In the wake of the recent era of civil rights reform, there have appeared some formal statements on the rights of patients. In 1973, the American Hospital Association issued a statement known as "A Patients' Bill of Rights" (see appendix A) in the expectation that its member hospitals would subscribe to it on behalf of patients. Many hospitals, in fact, did not adopt the bill while others gave it limited approval and low visibility.[12] In other words some hospitals quietly adopted the text but made it known only to key employees and did not post it publicly.

The bill was an attempt to enunciate in a formal way various principles regarding patient's rights, some of which many health-care institutions were already tacitly observing. Hardly anyone could quarrel with the clauses which state that the patient was entitled to "considerate and respectful care" and the right to "privacy and confidentiality." However, other clauses proved troublesome for some hospitals, especially in the prevailing atmosphere of malpractice litigation. The bill stated the patient had the right to "reasonable continuity of care" which was intended to prevent such things as dumping the patient on the curbstone for failure to pay the bill and to see that he did receive care from some source once he was discharged from the hospital. Some hospitals expressed trepidation over the possibility of lawsuits because of latitude in the interpretation of what constituted "continuity of care." The same kind of fears were expressed over the clause which made informed consent a right of the patient.

Possibly the most vexing clause was that which stated the patient had the right to obtain information from his physician about his diagnosis, treatment, and prognosis in language he could understand. Many hospital administrators expressed fear that this would require monitoring of the doctor-patient relationship which would, in effect, place the administration and the medical staff in "adversary roles." Yet, Leonard Bachman, a physician and Secretary of Health for the state of Pennsylvania publicly stated that the providers, hospitals, and physicians regarded the patients' rights movement in an adversary way and went on to add that the health-care providers in his state had blocked legislation by a very effective campaign against the patients' rights movement.[13]

Thus, many hospitals failed to adopt the bill as a policy because of the legal implications they envisioned. Other hospitals adopted the bill, stating that fear of litigation was not the proper reason for nonratification since the patient who felt wronged over his rights would take legal action whether the bill was a policy of the hospital or not. It has been estimated that only 30 percent of U.S. hospitals have adopted the bill. One state, Minnesota, made its adoption a legal requirement for hospitals and nursing homes, where it has to be visible for patients and staff.

Some have said that the bad hospitals would be the last to adopt the bill, reasoning that the better hospitals would be the first to adopt it or practice its principles. Most seemed to agree that the bill had a favorable effect on the protection and care of the patient. Continued pressure from consumer groups will likely provide the impetus for patients' rights legislation, with or without the help of the health-care professions. Meanwhile, there are other problems with existing rights declarations.

The bill itself and other similar statements suffer from three faults: they are provider-generated, they are sometimes self-serving and vague, and they lack an effective enforcement mechanism. Nevertheless, the principles of respect, privacy, confidentiality, and informed consent seem to have been well established and will be increasingly observed. However, the question of how much information the patient is entitled to obtain from his physician is still open-ended. In Massachusetts the patient may legally examine his or her hospital records and copy any portion of them; actually few patients know this or avail themselves of the privilege. Many good physicians feel that they should be the sole judge of what information the patient should receive, but this custom is often subject to abuse and may disappear under pressure from medical reformers and consumer groups. The federal government has insisted since 1974 that the basics of the bill be observed in skilled and intermediate care nursing homes serving Medicare and Medicaid patients and withholds payments if there is failure to comply. An influence as pervasive as HHS's could easily induce lawmakers to make the bill's basic provisions the law of the land.

Not everyone shares the convictions of those physicians who feel that they should be the sole judge of what information the patient should receive. Indeed, paragraph two of the Patients' Bill of Rights states that patients can reasonably expect to receive information about their diagnosis, treatment, and prognosis in understandable language. John A. McMahon, a lawyer and president of the American Hospital Association at the time it produced the bill, said that development of hospital medical staffs sensitive to patients' rights was one of the objectives of the association's malpractice prevention program for its member hospitals. He indicated that some of the hospitals' malpractice problems arose from lack of communication between patients and physicians.[14]

Patients want to communicate with their physicians and other medical providers, and many of them want a full disclosure of what is wrong with them and what is being planned for their care. This means the health-care profession must give up much of its traditional secrecy which many patients view as a device for obfuscation, if not deception. Furthermore, an informed patient is better equipped to cope with his medical condition and cooperate with the physician in the treatment process; a partnership or contract approach is hardly possible without good communication. Patients who do not establish good communications with their physicians simply do not respond optimally to therapy and are prime candidates for initiating malpractice actions.

There is a hauntingly familiar theme in the above; the medical profession should have led the reform drive for the establishment of patient's rights. Robert Chiles, who was not a physician, wrote one of the landmark articles on patient rights which appeared in a medical journal in 1967.[15] Chiles asserted that patients were entitled to certain basic rights, which he described. The ink was hardly dry before letters to the editor from irate physicians came pouring in. Several of them opined that since Chiles was "remote" from the world of medicine, he could hardly be an authority on the rights of patients. At this point the editor did a little opining himself, stating that no one who had ever been flat on his back as a patient in a hospital was remote from the world of medicine.

Chiles felt that the patient was entiled to privacy, to the right to express pain, and the right to the truth. These rights could also be seen as the right to respect, the right to be heard, and the right to be told; in short, the exercise of the Golden Rule would have sufficed. The Hippocratic legacy indicates that love, responsibility, and competence are expected from a practitioner of medicine, and the stewardship concept requires advocacy for the rights of the patient. This tradition and concept are compelling forces which should protect the patient, but they are too often unknown or ignored. The basic factor for the protection of the patient and his rights is caring or *philia*, which should bring about the needed reforms. Conversely, reforms made from fear of state intervention will ebb and flow with the iminence of the threat. In this context, *philia* is positive and enduring while fear is negative and transient. A mentality of advocacy must prevail in love for the continued protection of the patient.

A legal approach to the protection of patients and trial subjects suffers from limitations and, the patient or subject could be harmed or placed in jeopardy while the letter of the law is observed. Only the observance of medicine's ethical tradition will properly protect the patient or the experimental subject. The consistent application of the Golden Rule is better than a collection of laws, but until that happy state prevails, we appear to need the limited protection the law affords.

Theologian Paul Tillich reminds us that "'Person' is a moral concept pointing to a being which we are asked to respect as the bearer of a dignity equal to our own, and which we are not permitted to use as a means for a purpose, because it is purpose in itself."[16] This observation is certainly applicable to the person who is a patient or a trial subject.

CHAPTER **10** _____

MEDICINES OUT OF THE EARTH

_____

In the current confusion in our culture over the drug abuse problem, the physician is often turned to as an authority. Further, he is likely to be regarded as a person of integrity who is presumably free of any personal drug problem. All of these assumptions are unwarranted; in fact, there is clear evidence to the contrary. Increasing numbers of medical reports indicate that a substantial number of physicians have a personal drug problem and that improper prescribing and dispensing practices as well as negligent handling of dangerous drugs are widespread in the medical profession. This problem is compounded because most physicians delude themselves into thinking that they are more skilled in the use of these therapeutic agents than the facts would indicate. The entire problem area centering around the physician and drugs is an important ethical issue because of (1) the wide extent of the problem (2) the potential for control of the problem by the profession itself and (3) the distinct possibility that if drug abuse is not controlled soon, the medical profession and society in general will continue to deteriorate.

PERSONAL ABUSE OF DRUGS

We know that many physicians are impaired because of personal drug abuse or addiction. Such personal abuse may range from occasional indulgence to the point of being habituated or addicted. The actual drugs abused may be prescription drugs or illegal items such as marijuana or heroin. Abuse of any drug may affect competence or at least set a poor example for others; most people still expect physicians to be models of behavior. Problem drinkers in the profession form a significant portion of the drug abuse problem. The everyday stresses of working in medicine and the easy availability of medications make drug abuse an occupational hazard. An ancient medical tradition emphasizes the dangers inherent in self-diagnosis and treatment, but the profession seems to have a blind spot for the related problem of personal drug abuse. In a long range study Vaillant and his coworkers showed that the physician is much more prone to take mood-altering or psychoactive drugs than are the members of the general public.[1] Other reports have pointed out the hazards of drug dependency among physicians.[2] Use of marijuana and other illicit drugs by physicians is increasing.[3]

PHYSICIANS' CONTRIBUTIONS TO DRUG ABUSE BY OTHERS

Negligence in handling or storing drugs

Most physicians keep narcotics and other potent drugs in their homes and offices, as well as in their house-call bags. Rarely are these drugs as secure as they should be, and the doctor's bag, in particular, is a prime target for criminals or addicts. Usually several persons have access to the regular office stock and to many samples distributed by drug companies. Physicians' children have been poisoned by ingestion of mail samples delivered at home, and such a source is available for possible abuse by other family members. A considerable number of physicians in this country still keep large supplies from which they regularly dispense drugs to patients. Although the provisions of the so-called Dangerous Drug Act increase the physician's accountability, there are still many drugs with potential for abuse which are not listed as "controlled" substances under this act. The physician alert to this problem will keep his call bag in a safe place and secure his office drug supply by making one trusted employee the custodian and, as such, accountable by periodic inventory checks.

Handling drugs in a careless manner is another dangerous form of abuse. At a private clinic, I saw syringes loaded with various antibiotics and other medications placed in a tray without partitions in anticipation of the day's demands. The aides and nurses who dispensed these "shots" to patients told me they could easily tell the medications apart, but I could not, and I doubt that they could 100 percent of the time. Such a practice is extremely dangerous and would never be permitted by responsible supervisors.

The physician should avoid storing drugs at home and not allow the house-call bag to be a temptation to family members. One physician passing by the room of his teenage son late in the evening recognized a pattern of irregular breathing. On checking, he determined that the boy was suffering from a narcotic overdose and only prompt action saved his life. The boy had been using "street" narcotics which were normally "cut" or diluted by the distributor. On this occasion the boy had filched some morphine from his father's bag, and assuming the strength to be the same as his usual supply, had given himself a lethal amount. Accountability, security, and responsibility should be prime goals in the physician's handling of dangerous drugs.

Too liberal prescribing of psychoactive drugs

Patients and physicians alike are aware that many drugs affect one's state of mind, an effect which many find pleasurable and desirable. Many patients come to the doctor expecting to receive medications of this type and if it is not prescribed seek it elsewhere, usually from a more compliant physician—and such physicians are all too easily found. Herein lies a tragedy. Because some physicians will prescribe almost any drug the patient wants or will pay for, the good physician finds it difficult to practice good medicine. Why? Because when patients accustomed to getting what they want (or getting what a bad physician gives them) come to the ethical practitioner who gives only what is medically indicated, they leave his office disappointed and seek what they want elsewhere. Common examples of bad practice include routine use of antibiotics when not indicated (as for the common cold) and routine use of psychoactive drugs (sedatives or stimulants) as symptomatic treatment without trying to discover why the patient is worried, anxious, or depressed. Many undetected suicidal patients have visited a physician within a day or so of killing themselves.

Some years ago a survey disclosed that in Britian psychoactive drugs constituted some 15 percent of all prescriptions. It was theorized that this might be because Britons do not pay for most of their medications. Yet a recent survey in an American community revealed the comparable figure to be 17 percent, an amount considered excessive for this class of drugs.[4] For some four years I was associated with comprehensive health systems supplying health care to the indigent in both rural and metropolitan areas. My own survey of prescription writing at these facilities revealed similar figures, with an excessive use of tranquilizers. My own particular answer to this was to start a campaign against such zealous use among staff physicians, an approach that appears to be working. Small wonder that tranquilizers are a major portion of pharmaceutical industry production. There is a definite trend toward even greater use of psychoactive drugs; in the control of this trend, the physician is the *key* figure. The doctor's purpose, as a steward of health, is not to bring chemical nirvana to all his patients but to seek optimal ways of treating their problems.

Loose standards for the refilling of prescriptions

Conditions which lead to such misuse include the pressures of a busy practice, the profit factor for physician and pharmacy, the desire to please the patient, and inadequate knowledge of the dangers inherent in certain drugs or combinations of drugs. In the rush and bustle of a busy office practice, it is difficult to find time to answer the telephone, and so the harassed physician may delegate routine matters like the refilling of prescriptions to a medical extender or office aide. Thus, when the pharmacy calls requesting permission for a refill for a patient's prescription, this is often given by a nonphysician. Such a practice is usually limited to less potent drugs, but some classes of the so-called "controlled" substances (those with a high potential for abuse) can also be refilled by telephone. This is a poor practice; it can and does cause trouble. The physician should decide that he or she will personally approve the bulk of the prescription refills and that only one trusted assistant such as a qualified nurse or medical extender can approve refills from a definite list of less potent drugs. Regardless of who approves drug refills, they must be entered on the patient's record; all too often this information does not get charted, and there is little awareness of how much and what kind of medicine the patient is taking.

Certain disease conditions demand that the patient always have medications on hand; such conditions include heart disease, asthma, and convulsive disorders. In an emergency guidelines may permit small refills of such medications until the patient can see the physician for a recheck, but these guidelines must be carefully established so that misuse is difficult. Many physicians indicate on the original prescription whether a refill will be permitted and such a practice obviates mistakes and troublesome refill calls. Undoubtedly, medical negligence of the type described has helped to bring about some of the strict Federal Food and Drug Administration regulations which many physicians decry.

Inadequate experience and knowledge of pharmacology and therapeutics

This is perhaps the most pervasive and dangerous aspect of prescribing drugs. Most physicians believe that they have adequate knowledge of the drugs they use, but the evidence indicates otherwise. Physician educators of undoubted competence and experience such as Henry Dowling, Sir Derrick Dunlop, and Louis Lasagna in both professional and popular publications have extensively described the average physician's sometimes abysmal lack of knowledge of the drugs he or she uses, and the irrational ways in which they are used.[5] Included in this criticism are the house staffs of the hospitals of leading schools of medicine. Use of fixed combination drugs, antibiotics and others, continues to be a problem despite the fact that such drugs contain two or more agents in a fixed ratio. This does not allow the dosage to be tailored to the condition being treated, and authorities regard this as a dangerous practice. Fortunately, the introduction of new combination products seems to be decreasing, possibly because the FDA is demanding more rigorous proof of efficacy.

Antimicrobial agents also continue to be one of the most misused classes of drugs. For the most part this misuse takes the form of prescribing such an agent in the absence of an indication for it, using the wrong agent for the particular infecting organism, or using a toxic agent when a safer adequately effective alternate is available. As an example, the quantity of the antibiotic chloramphenicol that would be needed in this country, based on relatively narrow current indications, can be accurately predicted because of the current incidence of susceptible disease. However, the amounts actually used are greatly in excess of these predicted "legitimate" amounts, even though the drug may cause fatal blood dyscrasias.

Ampicillin, one of the semisynthetic penicillins, is widely prescribed by the profession without proper indications, largely because the pharmaceutical industry touted it as a broad spectrum antibiotic effective against a wide range of organisms. Actually, the proper indications for ampicillin are quite limited. One might hope that teaching medical centers would be free from such misconceptions, but one group of investigators found that ampicillin was widely misused at the prestigious Johns Hopkins Hospital.[6] A study of antibiotic use among a randomly selected sample of patients at Duke University Medical Center, showed that 64 percent of antibiotic therapy was not indicated or inappropriate in terms of drug or dosage.[7] For many years it has been considered poor practice to give tetracyclines to children less than eight years of age, and the American Academy of Pediatrics could find virtually no indications for its use in this age group. Yet in a study of children treated under the Tennessee Medicaid program, some four thousand children under eight years of age received tetracycline prescriptions, or some 7 percent of the total.[8] The main cause in these cases of misuse was lack of adequate knowledge of antibiotic therapy plus misleading claims from the pharmaceutical houses.

The U.S. Department of Health, Education, and Welfare issued a report in 1968 which confirms the above conclusions that the average physician lacks adequate knowledge of practical pharmacology.[9] The report noted—as has been confirmed by nongovernmental sources—that between 60 and 70 percent of physicians receive their first information on a new drug from the manufacturer, via medical journal advertising, direct mailing, or from the manufacturer's representative. The same HEW report stated that few medical schools instruct medical students in practical clinical therapeutics or pharmacology beyond a basic formal course early in their training. These basic courses, it should be noted, are usually theoretical rather than practical, and are offered before most students have had much opportunity to observe and work with patients. The HEW report urged that all medical schools teach practical therapeutics in a clinical orientation, that is, when actual work with patients begins, and continue to do so throughout the clinical years.

A related form of irrational drug use is polypharmacy, or what might be called the "therapeutic shotgun." Many so-called cough syrups persist as examples of polypharmacy.[10] Though unproved, the idea has long persisted in medicine that a combination of drugs is superior to a single agent. Whereas it is true that occasionally a combination of drugs is superior to a single agent by reason of synergism of action, this is not generally true. Most "shotguns" are of the over-the-counter variety—that is, they may be bought without prescription—but occasionally are found in prescription drugs as well. A difficulty in using a therapeutic shotgun is that the "shell" contains pellets of many kinds, of which only a few may be effective for the condition being treated; as a result too few of the correct ones ever reach the target.

Many of these nostrums were created before it became apparent to investigators that certain drugs may not only fail to augment the actions of other drugs with which they are combined but may actually impair or markedly reduce their efficacy. Knowledge of such drug interaction is growing daily among the pharmacologists but is still too limited among great numbers of those practitioners who provide the bulk of medical care in this country.

Another facet of improper drug use is that agents of little or no demonstrated value continue to be prescribed, despite recent corrective measures. The thalidomide disaster of the early sixties precipitated the Harris-Kefauver amendments to the Food and Drug Act in 1962. Prior to this, pharmaceutical houses had only to assure the government of the purity and safety of their products. The 1962 amendments required that drug houses now demonstrate effectiveness as well, including that of older drugs marketed prior to 1962. Currently, the FDA is reviewing the efficacy of all marketed drugs. Independent panels of experts rate drugs as "effective," "probably effective," "possibly effective," or "ineffective." Drugs in the last two categories cannot be marketed unless evidence of effectiveness is so substantial as to warrant reclassification.

This approach is to be commended, and we can only regret that the medical and pharmaceutical communities did not evolve it themselves. Indeed, when drugs of questionable value are finally withdrawn from the market because of FDA objections, there has often already been a storm of protest. Despite the loud grumblings of a vocal minority, organized medicine grudgingly admits the need for the new regulations. Warnings are increasingly heard that more regulations will be forthcoming unless effective self-regulation is practiced by the drug industry and the medical profession. When there was mounting evidence for the gross overprescribing of Valium and Librium, two popular benzodiazepine tranquilizers, the FDA threatened more stringent regulations if the abuse was not curbed. Since it was not, the FDA placed tighter regulations on the prescribing of these drugs. Time after time, when this has occurred, there has been a howl of outrage from some of the medical profession who had failed to curb their prescribing habits.[11]

One physician illustrates well some of these excesses in drug prescribing. Although he was a member of a multidoctor group doing primary care, this physician was pretty much of a lone wolf and had his own loyal following of patients, many of whom were recognized as being what has been described as "drug-seeking personalities." This physician had enormous dependency needs and was in the chronic grip of what I have described previously as the adulation disease. In his extreme anxiety to please his patients and be adored by them he would freely prescribe and refill all sorts of psychoactive and narcotic drugs. In addition, whenever a medical audit was performed on his patient records, it was apparent that his knowledge of pharmacology and therapeutic indications was extremely limited. There were many occasions where the possibility of drug interactions from his use of two or more incompatible drugs were noted. After several warnings from state and federal narcotics officers and well-meant remonstrations from his colleagues, he resigned from the group and continued his same style of practice alone. This physician has since been arrested by narcotics officers and charged with several violations. It is unfortunate that it took so long for such action for this physician has harmed the public and his profession. It is doubtful that patients accustomed to such indulgence can be educated to know what they should reasonably expect in the way of drugs from a competent and ethical physician.

A few generations ago only a few truly effective drugs were available to physicians, whereas today we have a prodigious array of potent drugs that are capable of producing great benefit or much harm. Moreover, we are now a drug-using society, and everyday drug use is an accepted norm. The media assail us daily with messages from the makers of analgesics, stomach acid neutralizers, laxatives, and so on. The medical profession does not escape this bombardment; even in the medical journals the hucksters are at work. Most physicians get their first information about a new drug from journal or mail advertising rather than from the medical literature itself. Although the AMA and other publishers of ethical medical journals allege that they screen advertising copy, it seems obvious that if they do screen it they are most lax about their standards. For example, the FDA has required several pharmaceutical companies to retract certain advertising claims which were carried in prestigious medical journals.

Drug advertising is not all bad; sales representatives and advertising perform a service by directing the attention of physicians to new products. However, it is virtually impossible to avoid the pervasive influence of medical advertising, and some of it is harmful if we rely on it as a principal source of information. Medical literature and professional meetings are preferred sources of balanced information on drug usage.

Since drug use is a way of life today, most patients come to the doctor expecting medication of some kind. It can be difficult to tell a patient that he or she does not need a pill or a shot; it is natural to want to be liked. It is an axiom with some practitioners that if you don't give the patient something, he will leave disappointed; hence, one should always prescribe something, perhaps people-pleasing pink placebo pills. Then, in fee-for-service practice it is easy enough to reason that the patient really needs an injection or prescription. In other cases, as in the Medicaid mills, no rationalization is needed for such practice; it is based on pure greed. In any case, the buck must stop somewhere in regard to unnecessary use of drugs. One of the traditions of the profession is to teach and so a good physician will teach his patients that not taking a drug can sometimes be as important as taking one, since medications can cause serious side effects, disease, or even interfere with healing. Consumer literature is stressing this point more and more, and a physician who is sparing in the use of drugs will find this practice increasingly accepted. Until such practice is more widely accepted, those of us with a conscience will have to endure those patients who are annoyed with us for not giving them what they want. In effect, the good stewards must suffer for the sins of the bad.

There is still another factor to be considered in the area of abuse. Faigel and others have noted that physicians generally feel that they have an absolute right to prescribe or use any drug they wish.[12] It's fairly obvious from published studies and personal observation that many physicians prescribe certain drugs despite inadequate expertise in the use of those agents. Faigel asks if we really and truly have the right to use any drug we choose and concludes that we do not unless we have adequate knowledge of the pharmacology and proper indications for that drug. He thinks violation of this principle is a breach of ethics. Expertise is needed if we are to help the patient and also if we are to avoid harm.

Many physicians use drugs inappropriately or use inappropriate drugs producing the problem area that has been called irrational drug use. As stewards of health, physicians must follow a tradition of competence and seek ways for maximizing rational drug use. A continuum of required courses in clinical therapeutics in the medical school years has been urged, but many school have not followed this recommendation. Required postgraduate hours in this area and continuing medical education courses seem essential if physicians are to improve this deficiency in their professional skills.

Peer review and audit committees are still another way to direct attention to the problem and press for solutions. Such committees attempt to assess the quality of medical care from written records. Reports in the literature have shown the value of such review processes as a way of improving general medical care and uncovering irrational drug use. One such report assessed the quality of hospital care for children. The committee found that misuse of antibiotics in the care of children was prevalent, and the drug misuse, particularly of antibiotics, accounted for some 80 percent of the instances of suboptimal care.[13] Voluntary means of increasing the practice of rational therapeutics should be sought by both the medical and pharmaceutical communities, or additional legal remedies will be forthcoming.[14]

Regulatory agencies, which offer one way of dealing with the problem, have come into existence largely because of the failure of the medical profession to take voluntary measures. The current Professional Standards Review Organization (PSRO) legislation is another example of regulatory measures passed by Congress because of medicine's failure to correct evident fraud and abuse by some medical providers in the federally funded Medicaid program. Although individual PSROs are made up of practicing physicians who are doing peer review on their colleagues, there are many who are bitterly opposed to such review. Yet the tradition of ethical medicine clearly calls for peer review for maintaining adequate professional standards, something that should have been done all along. If the PSRO concept doesn't work, the consequences should be obvious.

As for personal drug abuse, this is not just a matter of unprofessional conduct or even the deterioration of professional performance with resultant harm to others. Use of drugs, especially illicit ones, is often a group affair; a physician participating in such activities does violence to a professional, ethical tradition and to personal stewardship. It is bad enough when a physician becomes drug-impaired, but it is compounded when he says, in effect, "Look everybody, it's O.K. to do this, let's live it up!"

Physicians can never escape their obligation to set a good example for right conduct. Neither, as stewards, can they escape the responsibility of caring for their own bodies which are also a gift in trust. A detailed analysis of the causes for physician abuse or misuse of drugs is beyond the scope of this book. I have explored the root causes of drug abuse in our young people in an earlier publication.[15] Some of the causes of drug abuse discussed there apply equally to adults, including physicians. Lipinski has written a lucid article about motivations for drug abuse and points to a complex interaction between man, drugs, and society.[16]

There is only one place to begin treatment of this corrosive disease of the medical profession and that is within the brotherhood and by common consent. Self-discipline, even though obligatory, has not worked well in general, but if it does not work better in the future, physicians will be monitored entirely by lay officials of the government and that would be a tragedy. The tragedy, however, would be of medicine's own making, a point physicians should not forget. Physicians must expose incompetent and unethical behavior in colleagues, not with the motive of being punitive, but because they hope to correct and rehabilitate another human being worthy of this consideration.

The point is that the medical profession must always act to conserve and preserve competence within its ranks and offer a helping hand to those who need it. With particular respect to drugs, the physician must act in the best interests of his patient, as advocate, and as a good steward. The physician has an equal mandate to maintain competence in the entire field of drugs and therapeutics, to prescribe drugs rationally, and to obtain knowledge from reputable sources. In the book of *Ecclesiasticus*, there is a reference that states God has made medicines out of the earth for man's use and "he that is wise will not abhor them."[17] By the same token, as wise stewards, physicians should not abuse them.

CHAPTER 11

PHILIA *AMONG HEALTH PROFESSIONALS*

In addition to stating that medicine was a social science, the German pathologist Rudolf Virchow also made the perceptive observation that medicine was politics on a small scale. Now that the health care business is the second largest in the nation, it can hardly be called small, but it is certainly political. The classical Greeks viewed politics as one of the noblest of careers because it meant a selfless dedication to the improvement of the city-state. There is also another view of politics evoked by names like Tammany Hall, Pendergast, Teapot Dome, and Watergate which is characterized by motives of self-serving. Without knowing precisely which view Virchow had in mind in alluding to medicine as politics, I can suggest that he had something of each.

The political world of modern medicine is concerned, in part, with the relationships between physicians and other health-care professionals. Since medicine's avowed goal is the good health and competent care of the patient, inter-professional relationships should be used to work toward that goal.

All too often a state of harmony fails to exist within the healing professions; the problem is old but what is new is the emergence of many new types of health-care professionals. The medical scene is no longer dominated by the physician with support from the pharmacist and nurse; there is an array of nurses, nurse practitioners, nurses' aides, medical extenders, medical technicians, medical superspecialists, and a whole gaggle of administrators. I confess to being somewhat intimidated these days when I walk into a large medical center because I no longer feel at home there. I also feel mildly depersonalized, and I can indentify with patients who have expressed similar feelings. Nurses no longer wear caps for the most part and it's hard to figure out who's in charge. Nurses no longer answer the phone, that is the job of the ward clerk. A bevy of uniformed aides are busily going everywhere. The pharmacist no longer greets you at his window, the receptionist or the pharmacy technician might transmit your message to the pharmacist within his sanctum. Trying to find the pathologist in the teeming world of the laboratory or the radiologist in his electronic maze can be a frustrating experience. Want to see the administrator? I'm sorry, he's busy, would the assistant do?" And so on. I note that one person in 60 in this country is employed by a hospital, not just in the health-care field but in a hospital. Do we really need all those employees? Instead of trying to answer a baffling question, let's take a more detailed look at some of the more important characters with whom physicians interact.

INTERACTION WITH THE CLERGY

The clergyman is one of the least appreciated and under utilized health-care professionals. Since healing or restoration to wholeness often requires a multidemensional approach, the help of the clergy is sometimes required and often very helpful.

Many clergymen obtain training in the medical field in what is known as clinical pastoral education, which normally involves training within the hospital or medical center for varying periods of time. The training is aimed at increasing their counseling skills and their expertise in dealing with the stress associated with being hospitalized as well as situations involving death, the dying, and other occasions of grief. Such qualified clergy are far more comfortable and capable of dealing with these aspects of care than is the average physician and may contribute significantly to making a correct medical diagnosis. *A Storm, A Stress* is the title of a film produced by the AMA's now defunct Department of Medicine and Religion which portrays the participation of a clergyman in making the correct medical diagnosis in a patient. Additionally, qualified clergy help to relieve the anxiety or depression often seen in hospital patients. Since, in many cases, the clergy are not permitted to write notes on the medical record they must either verbally communicate with the attending physician, or a valuable contribution to the healing process may be lost. Qualified clergy should be asked to chart notes on patients' records.

In an effort to increase understanding and cooperation between physicians and religionists, the AMA created a Department of Medicine and Religion in 1962. Via local medical society sponsorship joint meetings were held between the two disciplines which most felt were productive. The department produced literature and films like the one mentioned above and sponsored many regional meetings for interchange between the two professions. (See chapter 4)

Despite laudable efforts to bring together the clergyman and physician, there is still a wide chasm between the two professions. A resident physician once remarked, "Who in the hell called *him?*" referring to the hospital chaplain who just entered the ward. To this unknowing physician, the presence of the chaplain signalled trouble, an omen of death like the circling of a vulture. Too many physicians view the clergy in a medical setting as intrusive, troublesome, and lacking in tact. Most physicians will tell you that they have had a bad encounter with a minister or rabbi who has gotten in the way of the medical personnel or perhaps alarmed the patient by a lack of tact. Yet, to balance this type of bad encounter there are many physicians who have had equally good ones. Part of the trouble arises from a misunderstanding on the part of both minister and doctor, due in part to the inept minister who has had little training and no specialized experience in clinical pastoral work. There are equally inept physicians in such circumstances. The clergyman's and physician's roles should be complementary, not antagonistic.

Granger Westberg is a minister with wide experience as a chaplain and educator in clinical pastoral training. In the past decade he has innovated a mode of care for people known as a church-clinic in which both physicians and specialized clergy work with each patient. He feels that such combined therapy has produced good results when medical treatment alone has failed.[1] If the church-clinic concept does nothing more than illustrate the importance of this joint approach to restoring wholeness it is still a significant contribution from which we can all learn. However, it is one model for providing comprehensive, holistic care.

It is important to understand the very personal nature of religious beliefs and values in the patient and to bear in mind the advocacy role in this regard. Patients entering a hospital are usually asked the name of their minister or their religious faith, but the physician should reinforce this point by asking the patient if he wishes to see a clergyman if one has not already been called. When I was delivering babies in general practice, I often baptized those who were likely to expire, not because of my personal feelings about the value of baptism but because this act often brought comfort to the parents. Needless to say, I knew my patients fairly well. Prudence is in order in such a well-meant act, since irate parents have sued hospitals when they found out their infants had been baptized without their permission.

Each practicing physician should get to know several of the local clergy well so that he can rely on their skill and competence in patient management. In large cities it is well to extend this relationship to ministers of the major faiths. Obviously, if there is a hospital chaplain he or she should be cultivated, and the chaplain should be encouraged to make rounds with the physicians and enter into discussions at medical meetings. One hears about the healing team concept from time to time, but it is a hollow phrase unless there is team work and team spirit. If there is an ethics committee, a clergyman should be on it. Medicine needs and should welcome qualified clergy as full partners if we are to practice the concept of total care.

THE PHARMACY PROFESSION

Friction and misunderstanding between medicine and pharmacy are probably as old as either profession. It is amusing to note that in 1550 an English physician named John Securis wrote that apothecaries should not "prescribe physic" and that their shops should be inspected from time to time by physicians. One pharmacist told me he had a stock answer for any customer who wanted his advice for what to take for a complaint. The pharmacist simply said, "I have an agreement with the doctor next door: I don't practice medicine and he doesn't sell drugs." While this may not strike you as humorous, it does touch on one trouble spot: most pharmacists do recommend nonprescription drugs and many physicians still dispense most of the medicine they prescribe. Many pharmacists are prudent enough to refer a customer to a physician if they suspect a serious condition. However, many physicians continue to sell medications even when there is a pharmacy in the area; it has been held that this is an unethical practice, and it can be. There is a built-in temptation to make more money here. The AMA does not recommend the practice unless there is no local pharmacy but curiously enough finds nothing unethical in physician ownership of a pharmacy "provided there is no exploitation of the patient."[2]

Pharamacists spend five or more years learning a great deal about pharmacology and pharmacy. Much has been written about whether pharmacy is a profession or a trade, since the bulk of pharmacists are cast in the role of merchants in the average retail pharmacy which sells everything from mouth wash to spark plugs. True, there are so-called ethical pharmacies which do nothing but dispense prescription drugs, but these are a minority. Because this image of the pharmacist as businessman is pervasive, the average physician often regards the pharmacist as a vendor of drugs who has no business questioning the doctor's prescriptions or prescribing habits. Since the lifeblood of the prescription department depends on the goodwill of the physicians who write prescriptions, the pharmacist is placed at a disadvantage. Still, the pharmacist is bound to check on any prescription which seems unusual in terms of dose, amount, how it is to be taken, or even the agent. Since many prescriptions are forged by addicts to obtain controlled substances, the pharmacy must occasionally check to see if the physician actually prescribed the drug.

Most physicians respond to this practice reasonably well, since they realize that nurses and pharmacists are required to do this checking, but occasionally there is an angry exchange during which the physician upbraids the pharmacist for daring to question his orders. The pharmacist is placed on the defensive, which can result in harm to the patient. A pharmacist who has had a bad experience with a given physician may be reluctant to check an unusual prescription which may have been written in error. Harry Shirkey is a well known pharmacologist noted for his quick wit and graphic lectures. Inevitably in one of his presentations a picture of a tombstone comes into view, reminding his audience of what can happen when mistakes are made in orders for medications.

It is easy to understand why some pharmacists react negatively to what they preceive as being a whipping boy or being treated in a patronizing manner or as an inferior by physicians. Now that there is little need for the individual preparation or compounding of prescriptions by skillfully mixing many ingredients, the pharmacist must often wonder why he spent five years in college learning such skills only to spend the bulk of his time counting pills and getting bad treatment.

Physicians must learn something about the training of the pharmacist and how to utilize him or her as a respected and valuable member of the health-care team. More pharmacists are being trained in clinical pharmacy and are knowledgeable in the area of drug interactions whereas many physicians are not. Many pharmacists keep a drug profile on each patient and when asked by the prescribing physician are pleased to comment on the possibility of a drug interaction if one exists. The pharmacist is also qualified to counsel the patient on the importance of following exact instructions of how and when to take the prescription and what to avoid taking with it. For example, the pharmacist can caution about the use of intoxicating beverages while taking tranquilizers. Pharmacists are capable of taking blood pressures and other vital signs, but they should have the support of the physician. If there is evidence that a patient is not well controlled by medications, then he or she can be referred back to the doctor.

In special circumstances pharmacists have been trained to function as "pharmacist practitioners" in which capacity they diagnose and treat common disease conditions. Further splintering of pharmacy in this direction is not advisable since the pharmacist's training is not a preparation for practitioner work; a fact one study indicated.[3] However, the field of clinical pharmacy is wide open as far as expansion and need are concerned.

In short, physicians should involve the pharmacist in patient care by utilizing his skills and recognizing his importance and contributions as a member of the health-care team. Pharmacists should participate in medical meetings at the encouragement and invitation of the physicians. The pharmacist is often the first point of contact for the patient who is seeking and in need of skilled health care. How the pharmacist handles that initial contact may be critical for the future health of that patient.

THE NURSING PROFESSION

Certain religious orders of monks and nuns began to care for the sick and needy in the hospices and hospitals established by early Christians. Over the years certain orders of nuns took the responsibility of providing nursing care to the sick. After the reformation, nursing declined in quality in those areas which were largely Protestant because they lacked the religious nursing orders. It was not until 1836 that the modern era of nursing began in Germany when Protestant sisterhoods of nursing were instituted; it appeared that the religious motivation was a necessary ingredient for survival of the art as it had been necessary for its institution in the first place. By the mid-eighteenth century these "lay sisterhoods" of nursing had been brought to England by a Quaker woman named Elizabeth Fry. What was new about the Protestant emphasis was the secular nature of the orders. The nurses were actively involved in worldly activities and were free to marry and lead outside lives but were dedicated to their work as a means of serving God. The distinctive caps which were formerly more visible in our nurses are a reminder of the religious orders from which they came as is the title of "sister" often used for English nurses.

Early nursing was relatively unskilled and consisted mostly of housekeeping and custodial functions for the patients with the giving of certain treatments or medications ordered by physi-

cians. Gradually the nursing role demanded more skill and training so that formal schools of training were established in several
hospitals before the twentieth century. A "trained nurse" was
one who had attended such a nursing school, while a "practical
nurse" was one who had taken up nursing without formal training. The registered nurse or R.N. and the licensed practical (or
vocational) nurse (L.P.N.) are the modern counterparts. The
R.N.s and the L.P.N.s and the nurses' aides were the principals of
hospital nursing services up to World War II.

For various reasons, some of which remain a mystery to me,
the nursing profession began an expansion after World War II
which is still continuing. In part, it was because nursing was
often an unappreciated role, and in the minds of some physicians
the nurses were still maids with mop buckets. Lack of apprecia-
tion certainly has made nurses determined to get more respect as
co-professionals with physicians. Medicine also became more
and more specialized and nursing felt the same impluse to diver-
sify, to specialize, and to acquire more status. In the postwar
years many universities instituted bacculaureate schools of nursing so that increasing numbers of nurses were graduated with
the degree of bachelor of science in nursing. Now we have
increasing numbers with master's degrees and even doctorates.
While all this is transpiring, we have a shortage of any type of
trained nurses in many of our institutions and many of them rely
heavily on L.P.N.s and aides. What has happened to nursing care?
If this lament has a familiar sound, it is because what has happened in nursing is a rough parallel of what has happened to
primary care in medicine. By primary care I mean the physician
with whom the patient has his first encounter, commonly visualized in this country as the kindly old general practitioner of
yesteryear.

After World War II, when the general practitioner began to
vanish, many American communities were without a physician
for the first time in memory. In the past decade we have seen a
resurgence of interest in primary care and the creation of a new
specialty, the family physician. However, another movement has
paralleled this which is the emergence of the so-called "mid-level
practitioners," the nurse practitioner and the physician's assist-

ant. Nurse practitioner schools have blossomed all around the country as one means of relieving the shortage of primary-care providers. Nurses entering this program are taught to take medicial histories and do physical examinations, to make elementary diagnoses and prescribe medications or treatments within established guidelines. There is no doubt that nurse practitioners perform well and are a tremendous help in certain contexts.

Now, however, the nurse practitioner concept is galloping away in the direction of specialization with family nurse practitioners, pediatric, and geriatric nurse practitioners, and perhaps even other nursing specialists. There seems to be no end in sight. This kind of superspecialization in nursing may well create the same imbalance which occurred within medicine so that we could have a maldistribution in both nursing and medicine. It seems that at least part of the nursing profession is bent on a totally independent existence apart from physicians. The nursing practice acts in most states recognize nursing as a separate profession, and many consumer boards are demanding that nurse practitioners be allowed to practice independently and do their own collecting of fees. I am concerned about the seemingly endless creation of new roles and the turning away from our basis obligations. Nurses are bound by the same Hippocratic legacy and *philia* as physicians and this will only be impeded by over-specialization. What seems needed is collaboration among health professionals rather than myriads of independent practitioners.

If this trend continues we will have competition among not only the various types of healing such as chiropracty, osteopathy, and allopathy but between the medical and nursing professions. And there will be those who will welcome such a development since such competition might bring down the cost of a medical encounter. Things don't have to go that way; there are cool and thinking heads in both prefessions who believe that there is a continued need for a closely-combined and collaborative approach to health care by both professions. We need nurse practitioners, and we need bedside nurses, just as we need medical specialists and generalists.

The time is overripe for stepping back and taking a good look at what is going on in both our professions. It may be that we can consolidate some gains and some roles and streamline the whole health-care operation insofar as medical providers are concerned. Creating more and more new roles is not the answer. It is time for physicians to realize that nursing has been neglected and unappreciated to some degree and that we should begin the business of building bridges between our separated isles.

A collaborative undertaking like the National Joint Practice Commission (NJPC) was a good example of how both professions can be mutually supportive in patient care. The NJPC was established as an interprofessional organization by the AMA and the American Nurses' Association and recently published a book which contains accounts of how certain physicians and nurses entered into joint practice with apparent benefits to all concerned.[4] In 1981, however, this joint venture was abandoned.

If we are to avoid any further partitioning of medical care, both professions should seek other areas in which they can be mutually supportive. It would help for both to remember that their relationship is interdependent and that each is necessary for any effective system of health care.

INTERACTION WITH MEDICAL ADMINISTRATION

If nurses are said to be essentially person-oriented and physicians disease-oriented (as some studies suggest) then medical administrators might be characterized as being "numbers-oriented." No wonder, either, since the medical administrator has daily concerns with quantifiable matters like square footage, depreciation, occupancy rate, cost-of-living index, cash flow, patient flow, numbers of physician encounters, and all those other figures involved with the business side of health care. An administrator also has to work within budgetary constraints and see that his or her organization does the same or risk fiscal disaster. Sensitivity to financial matters often amounts to a preoccupation that is often a source of difficulty to other health-care personnel.

Most physicians, by contrast, lack an adequate amount of financial sensitivity and from the administrative point of view often make unreasonable demands for more space or equipment without economically utilizing the existing facilities. Physicians are accustomed to having a highly expensive and complicated workshop provided them without cost in the form of a hospital or clinic for the purpose of treating patients from which services they earn fees. These divergent points of view on fiscal matters often lead to friction, hostility, and subsequent breakdown of what must be a team effort. The result is that the administrator often regards the physicians as "spoiled brats" who contribute little to the total effort except criticism and yet earn a handsome income. From the physicians' point of view, the administrator is a demanding martinet who insists on running a tight ship without a proper understanding of the problems and responsibilities of the officers and crew.

Obviously both physicians and administration provide health care, since the physicians would be hard put to provide patient care without proper facilities and staffing. In the complex inter-dependency of modern health care, the physicians simply need the help of the administrator as captain of the support team. Knowledge of each other's needs and problems can help to buffer the abrasive zones. Physicians need to become more involved with fiscal planning and take some initiative in keeping down the costs of health care, while administrators need to know more about the problems and descision-making facing the medical staff in their daily interactions with patients. In short, adminis-trators need to know more about people as patients and how physicians care for them.

Perhaps it might help if physicians could view medical adminis-trators as they would their own stockbroker or banker. In other words the administrator is actively looking after the doctor's interests as well as the patients' by making a health-care facility possible for both. This view might ease the adversary overtones in the administrator-physician relationship. Working together to cut down the costs to the patient and provide better care all around requires *philia* and good stewardship from everyone on the health-care team.

The foregoing discussion may strike you as facile and simplistic or even obvious. All we have to do is love one another and understand each other's profession so we can work as a team and everything will be just peachy. That's precisely one of the points I am trying to make; the formula for improving health care interrelationships is not complicated; it's putting the formula into practice that is difficult. Early in our careers we must sensitize ourselves to the need for close collaboration with our colleagues and constantly work at staying sensitive and seek ways to understand one another's work.

There is a course run by students in the health-care field to improve interprofessional relationships between health care personnel. At Columbia University students from four health professions, medicine, nursing, occupational therapy, and physical therapy initiated a course designed to improve knowledge of one another's training and skills with the larger objective of preparing themselves to work within a team context.[5] This approach contains the basic ingredients for improved interprofessional understanding.

Much more could be said about the relationships between physicians and physical therapists, occupational therapists, medical technicians, and even housekeeping personnel. However, many of the points made earlier could apply equally well to all members of the health team. Basically, it's important to know there is a team concept in which all must be included and that everyone's contributions are necessary and appreciated.

PHYSICIAN TO PHYSICIAN

Poor though interprofessional relations may be at times, there is another troubled area that is even more disturbing; this is the area of the relationships that too often prevail between physicians.

Until relatively recently there has been little to guide physicians in their conduct toward one another. The Hippocratic Oath does express the idea of brotherhood for physicians, but this appeared to be the norm for members of a tightly knit cult of healers. Regardless, the medical profession has taken up the spirit of the oath, and it is regrettable that the brotherhood motif has not been more widely accepted. There is a fairly standard professionalization process through which all physicians must go, and this should be a unifying force for improved relationships. In any case the ordinary rules of courtesy and kindness ought to prevail between physicians as professionals.

We have seen how various physicians through the centuries have formulated codes of behavior or statements of belief for their own guidance and that of others. Such attempts were sporadic and too often did little to influence the behavior of what has been heterogenous group of "healers." It was a recognition of this chaotic state of affairs in the medical world that led Percival to formulate his Code of Ethics in 1803 in London. For the most part his code set down rules of conduct between patient and physician or between physicians and was largely a form of etiquette or medical good manners for that time. Percival stated that physicians should avoid "officious interference" in a case under the care of another physician but left no doubt that there were occasions in which negligence or incompetence in another physician were so serious that the ethical physician had no choice but to make a "spirited interposition." Whatever its faults, the code was a landmark in emphasising the importance of good intraprofessional conduct.

Both history and experience tell us that physicians are not always kind and considerate to one another. Many of the medical giants, past and present, have been abrasive, rude, and irascible toward their colleagues. On the other hand, other medical notables suffered greatly at the hands of their colleagues who virtually ostracized them. Paracelsus seems to have fit the first type well, while Semmelweis, the discoverer of the cause of childbed fever, represented the second type. Most people are inclined to overlook the bad behavior of the medical giants simply because of their medical contributions, but there are too many physicians who hate or resent certain colleagues and often react in undesirable ways.

The reasons for such poor conduct toward a colleague are often complex but sometimes quite simple. It seems clear, however, that in many cases the physician who initiates the bad feelings is absolutely blind to his own real feelings and motivations and has built a protective shield via a process of rationalization. Certain emotions like greed, envy, fear, suspicion, and feelings of insecurity all contribute at times. Medicine is a demanding and fearsomely tough business at times, dealing every day with decisions involving life and death, and some physicians need thick insulating ego defenses while others are blessed with lesser needs. Famed trail lawyer Melvin Belli observed that many individual doctors seemed to be dedicated men who were concerned for reforms in medicine, but that in a convention or other assemblage they acquired a callous mob psychology that took over the individual physician's ethics and honesty. He also stated that lawyers displayed the same phenomenon.

There are certain professional diseases which affect the behavior of physicians toward one another, and one of these was discussed earlier as adulation disease. We also see the martyr syndrome in its pure form but commonly mixed with the adulation disease. Diagnosis of the martyr syndrome is made with the observation that a given physician is working himself to death, a fact he will commonly affirm because he needs to feel martyred. Diagnosis is further confirmed by observing that the "patient" will refuse to take time off for rest or get an associate or partner to share the burden. Men in the grip of MS often behave in strange or inappropriate ways toward their peers, but they are commonly adored and pitied by their patients. Another disease complex commonly seen in surgeons is known as omniscient wonder worker sickness. It's really a variant of the old-time authoritarian physician, but whatever it's called, the etiology is the same; excessive need for ego defenses.

Everyone needs ego gratificaton to some degree, but this need should not cause harm and mischief to the profession and patients. If physicians could be trained to recognize the unhealthy or destructive ego defense modes in themselves, they might develop more desirable modes of defense which would lessen harm to themselves and their fellow physicians. Many physicians are guilty of being critical of another's performance in what often constitutes malicious medical gossip. But when such physicians are asked to make a formal complaint against another physician or testify against him or her in a hearing, many will avoid doing so. A mechanism which operates here and which was mentioned earlier is the ability of most physicians to place them-

selves in the other's shoes in such a case and honestly ask themselves whether they couldn't have made the same mistake or
committed the same negligent act. Clearly, in certain cases physicians can put themselves in the other's place even though this
mechanism may prevent needed testimony from being heard.

My question is, if we can make this projection in certain cases
why can't we do it in others? Why, for instance, can't we be more
tolerant of the physician with a style of practice different from
ours, or toward a new physician in the area who needs to earn a
living as much as we, or even of the physician whose ego needs
differ from ours? In ruminating over this section and the questions it raised, I thought of some "case histories" of which I had
knowledge and which might serve to illustrate some of the points
I have tried to make.

(A) A young physician was hired by an older physician to help
him in a busy practice founded by the older man. As soon as the
younger man began to attract a following of patients the senior
physician began to openly criticize the abilities of the new man to
the patients who were expressing satisfaction with the new man.

In this case it is obvious that the older physician was jealous of
the popularity of his young colleague, an emotion he did little to
hide. The older man was overworked and bordering on senility;
he was often forgetful and childlike. He was affluent and could
easily afford to retire. In a case like this, it is possible that other
medical colleagues could have persuaded the senior physician to
retire with a little nudging from the state licensing board, since it
was recognized that the older man's competence was becoming
impaired. This was an opportunity for situation ethics to prevent
further harm to the community and save a disintegrating
practice.

(B) Dr. X, a physician with a large practice, induced another
physician, Dr. Y, to move from a distant city and join him in
practice because X could no longer handle his practice alone; he
was exhausted and needed help. X told Y that he need not worry
about expenses at first since he needed help badly and only after
Y developed his own practice would there be a sharing of office
expenses. Y moved his family to the new area but within a few
days X collapsed from fatigue and asked Y to handle his practice

until he could recuperate. After a few weeks, the rejuvenated X returned to his practice and told Y he was no longer interested in any type of association and that Y would have to make his own arrangements elsewhere.

Other physicians in the area were well aware that X had followed a similar pattern of behavior with several other temporary associates. However, they did nothing to prevent a further recurrence and they failed to tell Y that X had a bad history with associates. In the traditional spirit of compassion and concern, the other physicians could have dissuaded X from future actions of this kind and tried to make him understand that he could not tolerate an associate in his practice because he suffered from the martyr syndrome. In the same spirit the new physician should have been informed of what had happened to previous associates of X before he agreed to the association. Our ethical heritage tells us that there are times when we must be our brother's keeper. (C) I once wrote another physician asking for information about a surgical procedure he had performed on a patient who was currently under my care. When several weeks had passed without a reply, I contacted the surgeon by telephone. Yes, he remembered the patient clearly enough, but the reason he had not responded was that the patient still owed him an unpaid balance, and he would be pleased to send a report after the account was settled! I was so surprised by what I considered a crass commercial attitude on the part of this doctor that I could only make a banal remark or two and then hung up. After a little reflection, I wrote this surgeon a note saying that I understood his feelings even if I did not agree with his actions and that I presumed we had both taken the same oath on graduation from medical school. I added that it was quite likely I would not be paid for my services either, since the patient was unemployed but that we as physicians had some obligation to care for patients with financial problems. Shortly thereafter I received the operative report I had requested. I think my admission of similar feelings rather than expressing moral indignation probably persuaded the surgeon to relent. Colleagues who sincerely try to reason with an errant brother physician must generate an atmosphere of empathy and helpfulness.

(D) A pediatrician hospitalized an infant with an intestinal disorder which remained refractory to treatment. He was aware that the family had formerly been under the care of another physician in the area. Despite all the customary diagnostic and therapeutic approaches the illness continued. The pediatrician called in another pediatrician as a consultant who reviewed the case and could suggest nothing further but felt that the condition would resolve in time. Suddenly the pediatrician was informed by the parents that he was discharged from the case because he had lied to them about the condition of their child and that their former physician would be assuming care of the case. The next day the parents filed a formal complaint against the pediatrician through the hospital medical staff. An ad hoc committee of staff physicians reviewed the entire case with the pediatrician in the presence of the parents and could find no evidence of mismanagement or misrepresentation. The father apologized to the committee and the pediatrician for his unfounded complaint. The committee chairman then asked the father if anyone had suggested that he make such a complaint and was told that his former physician had strongly urged this course of action.

In the above case the parents cannot be blamed; we all anguish over the continued illness of a loved one. In their distress they turned for help to their former physician who let his personal feelings dominate his ethical obligations. Unknown to the parents but well known to the medical staff was that their former doctor suffered from adulation disease in its chronic form. This man could have resumed the care of the infant without incident, but he chose rather to indict a colleague who had, in his thinking, stolen a patient from him. The committee acted laudably in their investigation of the complaint without bias and in exonerating the pediatrician; they also acted commendably in pointing to the real cause for the complaint so that everyone concerned was made aware of the truth. This is how it should be; committees should work without guise and provide access to people with complaints.

(E) A community hospital was staffed only by specialists who finally decided to establish a residency training program in general practice. The thinking of the medical staff was that they would provide a learning experience for a young physician who would provide them with help in the care of private patients. One trainee was interested in practice in the community after the completion of his training but was told by the residency committee that generalists were not accepted on the medical staff. One of the staff physicians who became aware of this inconsistent attitude wrote to the regional director of the training program to point out this exploitation of trainees to the benefit of the medical staff. When other members of the medical staff learned of this correspondence, they launched a bitter attack against the physician who had acted out of conscience but who, in their view, had betrayed them. The attack took the form of trying to prove that the complaining physician was incompetent and uncooperative. Happily, this attempt failed and the hospital board ultimately pressured the medical staff into giving hospital privileges to general practitioners.

It should be clear by now that physicians are as apt to be unaware of their true feelings and motives as anyone. In the above case the medical staff clearly hoped to gain more than they gave; they needed the help a resident physician could provide, but they were unwilling to let this physician remain in the community to compete for patients. Their great anger and overreaction was due, in part, to the fact that they had not faced the true facts in this case and so lashed out at the one they perceived as being the troublemaker. Hospital boards must be more than a rubber stamp for the medical staff; in many cases they can cause the medical staff to take a good inward look at itself and initiate right action.

(F) A physician wishing to open an office at a new location checked with the local medical society to see if it would be appropriate to place a notice in the local newspaper of his intended opening. He was told there would be no objection, and he subsequently placed a notice in the local weekly newspaper. Within hours the newcomer was called by an official of the local medical society who informed him that there had been a complaint from a local physician that the new man was unethically advertising! The sequence of events was explained to the official to his satisfaction. The new physician subsequently learned that the complainant was a physician who was heavily involved with gambling and other questionable business activities and who was on the verge of bankruptcy.

In the foregoing case it seems pretty clear that the complaining physician was influenced by the emotional strain of his impending financial ruin. His resentment of new physicians was aberrant and unjustified for he viewed them as competitors who were responsible for his downward course rather than looking to himself as the reason. This is further reflected by his charge of "unethical advertising" while he was engaged in certain illegal activities himself. Again, the medical community was aware of the questionable activities of the complainant, but no corrective action was offered.

What can be done to improve relationships between physicians? Clearly, medicine needs men and women of good will who are reasonably free of mental aberrations and are capable of working within the context of *philia* love. The selection process for medical students is one area where more sensitive screening might be done.

Perhaps premedical students could be required to take awareness or sensitivity training so they could be more knowledgeable of the traps that medical practice can sometimes spring and of how their personalities affect others. It would seem appropriate to acquaint students with the principles of situation ethics and of how situationism would operate toward physicians as well as patients. Case histories could be presented and discussed. Looking back over the years, I can see how such training would have helped me. Why should physicians not practice preventive medicine on themselves? Why not continue this awareness training in medical school and as a part of continuing education in the practice years? Such programs do exist now but more are needed.[6]

The medical community must also take corrective action against those physicians who have a chronic history of bad relationships with their peers. The medical community is usually well aware of the problem physician but often does nothing to help. Such offending physicians can be offered help in love rather than punitive measures. Oftentimes counseling by colleagues of good will is enough to cause a change for the better. Far too often these deviant physicians are ignored until they become such a problem that drastic action is required.

The Hippocratic legacy of brotherhood indicates the relationship physicians should have with one another. The traditions of *philia* and responsibility apply equally to colleague, patient, and society. The practice of medicine is becoming more complex with many new health professionals making up the health-care team. If the team is to function effectively, it will require application of the Golden Rule among physicians and between physicians and other members of the team. Physician, heal thyself: this admonition is basic to professionalism.

CHAPTER 12

CAN THE MEDICAL EDUCATORS LEARN?

It is curious that in the current interest in the teaching of ethics in medical education so little attention has been given to the corporate ethics of the schools themselves. Like Caesar's wife, they have been above reproach but like Caesar's wife, they may deserve reproach. Medical schools are uniquely situated in our society for it is only through them that one may become a physician today. Furthermore, all medical schools accept public funds to some degree. For these reasons alone the medical schools should have some public accountability, but there are several other ethical implications that immediately arise: How are students selected and trained? Does the quantity and quality of those trained reflect the needs of our society? How is competence assured in those who are graduated as physicians? How is the faculty selected?

Although the primary goal of a medical school must be to produce physicians, the schools themselves have long insisted on the triple goals of education, research, and service. These goals are essential and ought to be interrelated: proper training requires that students see quality medical care being provided to the community and also participate in providing such care; they must also see medical research performed and understand the importance of furthering medical knowledge. In addition, no medical school may escape the ethical implications of selecting and training its students. For a better understanding of this process, a brief historical survey is needed.

Until the second decade of this century, medical education was generally in a state of chaos in this country. I described earlier how the reorganized AMA commissioned the Carnegie Foundation for the Advancement of Teaching to study the medical education system in this country and Canada, and the result was the epochal Flexner report in 1910. This report led to the closing of bad schools and hastened the development of a standard medical curriculum in the surviving schools. These surviving schools all stressed a firm foundation of basic science relevant to medicine, and most of them had a university affiliation. Other consequences of the Flexner report were discussed in chapter 5, but a few are highly significant for our present discussion. The same number of applicants for medical school were now looking at a greatly reduced number of openings. Standards for admission were raised, and there was an increasing emphasis on a scientific background. Within a short time all medical schools required a college degree or a minimum of two years of college work for admission. Medical schools become more and more preoccupied with the scientific aspects of medicine leading to what might be called the "lab-coat mentality" since it became increasingly important to wear a long white coat to remind everyone that the wearer was, first of all, a scientist.[1]

The events leading to the lab-coat mentality are understandable, but in their increasing preoccupation with medical science, the medical schools neglected the human side of medicine. During the period around World War II, it became increasingly apparent that more doctors were needed, and there was a gradual increase in the number of applicants. Admission committees became ever more selective, taking only what they perceived as the best students. Over the years a Medical College Admission Test (MCAT) was gradually evolved from a brief essay-type test to a formidable objective-type instrument which probed the cognitive aspects or knowledge of the applicant, especially in the mathematical and scientific areas. Another criterion became important; the Grade Point Average (GPA) of the applicant's preliminary college work.

Despite some sentiment for medical students who had been broadly trained in the humanities, it became increasingly clear to the post-World War II medical school applicants that high MCAT and GPA scores plus a heavy background in science was what the admissions committees really wanted. Fierce competition has gradually developed for the limited number of openings, even though the total number of first-year slots has roughly doubled since World War II. Occasionally premedical students have not hesitated to cheat on examinations or sabotage the academic work of their "competitors," a condition that has not escaped the notice of the media.[2] Applicants or their parents have paid out several thousand dollars in some cases to legislators when admission to a state medical school was involved or made "contributions" directly to the school. The news media carried many stories about this problem and it was the subject of the *Weekend Show* #36 carried on the NBC network for August 6, 1977 (transcript available).

All of these factors have had some questionable effects on medical students, many of whom become quite cynical, while a fairly constant percentage drop out of school largely for emotional reasons. Not enough is known about the long-term effects of excessive stress during the professionalization process, but clearly it is stressful and in some cases does cause harm to the student. Less clear is what the effects of such academic stress might be on the manner in which the future physician conducts his practice; additional studies are urgently needed. Although some stress is necessary to develop a certain amount of toughness which all of us need to survive and even to excel, excessive stress during the professionalization period is harmful, and the medical education community has an ethical obligation to study this matter thoroughly and take appropriate action.

I propose to describe what may be a typical applicant for medical school as conditions now exist and sketch the progress of that applicant through his training until he enters practice. This strategy might delineate the way things are, and how they might be improved. Our typical Joe or Jane Applicant may come from a white, urban, reasonably affluent, upper-middle-class family, which is usually able to afford the costs of medical school. The applicant is usually strongly achievement-oriented and has learned to survive and excel in a highly competitive educational jungle. He or she has had at least three years of college work stressing science and mathematics. The applicant often believes that the end justifies the means, and may, therefore cheat, lie, or even damage the work of his peers to keep his own GPA within acceptance levels. In short, our prototypical applicant is scientifically trained and Machiavellian.[3] Little more is known about this applicant to the typical admissions committee.

Our applicant presents himself to the admissions committee ready to swear that only the purest of motives bring him to this point and that all he wants to do is serve humanity.[4] The admissions committee members note that our applicant has high MCAT and GPA scores, has majored in science, and has the normal letters of recommendation from two physicians who are alumni of the school. A typical reference from one of the applicant's undergraduate instructors reads somewhat as follows: "Joe Applicant was in my course 201 (Differential Equations) and ranked second in a class of 32. I did not know him personally. He is a superior student."

Now the admissions committee knows that Joe is going to have two hard years of courses that are as difficult as Differential Equations was and on the basis of his scores and background knows that he has an excellent chance of getting through the basic science years and into the clinical years where failure is almost unknown. Joe's hair has been cut short and combed, and he wears a tie for this special occasion. The committee puts his folder into the select group already screened, and he is ultimately admitted.

Joe (or Jane) Applicant matriculates and enters the world of medical science. However, for the first two years he often sees little of medicine as it has appeared in cinema and on television, and although he visualizes himself as a graduate student, he sits daily in a classroom that differs little from that which he attended in high school, and he is little more than a name to the instructor, whom he perceives as being detached and impersonal. The fact is that few instructors in medical school at any level have had any training in educational methods, and many of them accept teaching as a sort of "medical KP" they must endure to keep their research projects going. This is one role model which Joe and Jane see far too often.

The clinical instructors are often no better as role models. Although they are "real doctors" many of them have medical research projects in highly specialized fields, and they may have little interest in teaching. The teaching takes place in a modern medical center offering tertiary or highly specialized care for many rare and esoteric diseases; in other words, the hospital patient population is anything but typical of what one encounters in the everyday practice of primary care medicine. Joe and Jane do not know this, and they see that the peak achievement of medicine is to stalk through the hospital corridors wearing a lab coat, treating rare disease and/or doing research. There are ambulatory clinics attached to the hospital, but these are known as the "pits" or by whatever derrogatory term is currently popular and are largely viewed as an exercise in futility since most of the patients have chronic disease and others are often referred to as "crocks" or "psychoceramics."[5] It bears emphasizing that the patient populations in these clinics may also be far from what one would encounter in average practice, but somehow this fact is not established. In short, the average university medical center, with its associated ambulatory clinics, is not providing an accurate reflection of what the general practice of medicine is like.

There are further difficulties for Joe and Jane. They learn from a few instructors that prevention is preferable to treatment of disease, but what they see in the hospital wards and clinics are the end results of a lack of prevention. One would like to think that such a state of affairs would stiffen the resolve of medical students to practice preventive medicine as much as possible, but it appears that many students become apathetic about the value of preventive methods since they seem so seldom utilized. Only the more perceptive students will figure out that the majority of patients seen in such medical centers are poor and have only known crisis care; and believe that they can't go to a doctor unless they are sick. It is equally possible for many students to dismiss the poor as being disinterested in prevention, and hence the sense of futility referred to earlier is only heightened.

So far Joe and Jane have had a premedical education with a major in science, and two years of medical school with virtually all medically-related science courses. Now in the third and fourth years, where they are learning "clinical science," the emphasis is still on science within the pervasive atmosphere of the lab-coat mentality. Where do these medical students learn about people, the person in the body, the human side of medicine, and holistic concepts of care? These aspects of medicine can be learned from one's preceptors or from material presented in didactic courses but ideally should be learned from a pervasive atmosphere of humane medical practice. However, in many medical schools it is a matter of chance whether Joe or Jane has adequate exposure to the human aspects of medicine.

By the time Joe is ready to graduate from medical school, he has decided to become a surgeon and will probably settle on one of the surgical specialties. In the wards and clinics of the medical center, Joe has perceived that ambulatory care and primary medical specialties are not held in high esteem. From his point of view the family practice residents were never in the mainstream of hospital medicine where he felt the real action to be. Also, Joe has had no advisor to guide him, and he does not realize how overcrowded a field surgery is nor how much need there is for primary care physicians in many underserved areas. I am not arguing here for the relative merits of primary care or surgery, but I want to point to what is all too often a skewed or unrealistic presentation to the student of what constitutes medical practice.

I must leave Joe and Jane at this point but I must make it clear that these prototypes are not distortions but frighteningly real because all of the characteristics I have assigned to them have been documented in medical students. Yes, there are humane and concerned medical students who do want to serve society, but for reasons I hope to make clear, such students are not numerous enough. The admission process may selectively eliminate many of them. Most of the medical school applicants come from backgrounds similar to our Joe and Jane and the majority of medical students are still entering specialty training rather than primary care fields which are generally considered to be general or family practice, pediatrics, and internal medicine. Underserved areas continue to be underserved, and the poor continue to get the worst or the least medical care. Meanwhile, GMENAC predicts a surplus of physicians by 1990.

In one study, a group of resident physicians in their first year of postgraduate training were followed for 7 years from 1968 to 1975. Results indicated that these young physicians were attracted to nonprimary care specialties in greater numbers than were physicians in the past and were continuing the trend away from rural practice locations.[6] Another study of the practice plans of students entering medical school revealed that some 70 percent preferred primary care and the majority preferred small or mid-size cities for location.[7] This apparent paradox may reflect a change in the few years separating these studies but, more ominously, it probably means that once entered in the medical milieu, like Joe and Jane, medical students are influenced away from primary care and rural locations; areas where they are most needed.

Having followed Joe and Jane to this point I propose to retrace this course and see what is being done to remedy some of the faults noted and what more might be done within the medical education continuum. A medical school has strong control over whom it will admit, considerable control over what and how they are taught, and increasing contact and influence with those who enter postgraduate training (the residency years), as well as having an increased contact and responsibility within the field of continuing medical education. I propose to examine all of these areas in turn.

THE SELECTION PROCESS

Ours is a highly competitive society, and our children are placed in competitive roles even before they enter grade school. In the case of medical students the process continues and intensifies in the premedical years. If we can agree that this is not the optimal preparation for future physicians, then what might be done to change it? We probably won't be able to change the competitive mentality much for many years to come, and I won't debate the desireability of limited competitive spirit; I am concerned about the excesses. We can develop alternative methods for selecting medical students based on the applicants' personality characteristics in addition to their cognitive abilities as measured by academic scores and special tests.

Weingartner has made ten suggestions for improving the selection process that could be readily implemented if the higher education community could agree to them.[8] He recommends:

1. The grade point average (GPA) should be computed only for the applicant's required science courses. This should encourage the taking of courses in non-science fields.

2. Medical schools should require either an undergraduate major in some field other than biology, biochemistry, or chemistry such as the humanities and behavioral science or evidence of a "significant" number of courses in these latter areas.

3. The pre-medical major should be eliminated. This would permit more flexibility in preparing for medical school.

4. Assure a broad education in applicants by requiring a bachelor's degree.

5. An expanded Medical College Admission Test that would include writing of an essay.

6. Instead of selecting students on their absolute GPA, schools should establish a *minimum* GPA so that once past that hurdle the application would be judged on its merits other than an absolute, ranked score.

7. A formula should be devised to equate the GPA's coming from different colleges since there is a vast difference in what they represent in terms of scholastic ability.

8. A scheme that would offer early acceptance to a medical school pending completion of the student's requirements for the bachelor's degree. This would enable a student, once accepted, to pursue a broad education in his college course rather than pursuing admission to a medical school.

9. Improved representation on the admission committee of medical schools. The author would have a faculty person from an "arts-and-science" department on the admission committee which would increase credibility in applicants that a broad education was important.

10. Each medical school should declare to the world that it will preferentially admit broadly educated applicants rather than machines which crank out high grades.

The author feels that these steps are possible but admits that it will take determined effort to achieve consensus for their acceptance. These recommendations deserve trial.

The path to alternative methods is thorny at best. Part of the problem is that (1) we are not entirely sure of what personality characteristics make better physicians, and (2) we have only recently begun the search for valid and reliable methods for measuring such personality traits. Although this is a challenging and intriguing field in which much needs to be done, the progress has been painfully slow.

Another reason for lack of progress is that admissions committees have been slow to change, reflecting the resistance to change that exists in many if not most medical schools. Academic freedom is no guarantor of open minds. For example, although the majority of dropouts from medical school are for emotional reasons, I know of only a few schools which require a psychiatric or psychologic screening. Efficient test instruments exist, like the Personality Orientation Inventory or the Meyer-Briggs Type Indicator (MBTI), which are easy to administer and score, but acceptance has been slow. Yet, candidates for the seminaries of many religious denominations are required to have a psychiatric examination. The MBTI has been given to applicants at the Eastern Virginia School of Medicine for several years but these have been used only for research and not counted in the selection process. Now the Personality Orientation Inventory is used because it is felt to be a better instrument by the researchers, but these scores still have no bearing on the admission decision. The fear was expressed that a rejected applicant might litigate, claiming discrimination on the basis of his or her personality testing. The Association of American Medical Colleges (AAMC) initiated a project in 1973 known as the Medical College Admissions Assessment Program (MCAAP). This project had the close cooperation and support of the medical schools and other groups concerned with medical college admission procedures and the search for better selection methods. There was general agreement of the need for (1) cognitive and (2) noncognitive or personality assessment of applicants and (3) establishment of clinical performance criteria by which the medical skills of students could be evaluated in the clinical years of school.

The old standard MCAT assessed the cognitive skills and basic knowledge of an applicant in the scientific, mathematical, and general areas, but it had many limitations. For example, correlation between MCAT scores and medical school performance was poor; a better predictor was needed. Hence, a new MCAT was devised and first given in 1977 and is by now fairly well standardized. In addition to most of the previous areas tested, it probes the analytical and problem-solving skills of the applicant. Results of studies on the new MCAT indicate that it is a very good predictor of academic success in the first year of medical school.[9]

The noncognitive program has not made much progress. Ambitiously conceived, it was to develop an assessment package which would be available to medical schools for collecting data on seven personality qualities of applicants: compassion, coping capabilities, decision making, interprofessional relations, realistic self-appraisal, sensitivity in interpersonal relations, and endurance in physical and motivational areas. Appropriate research groups and individuals were recruited to initiate the project while funding was being sought. It is a sad commentary on our times that some funding agencies refused to finance the program, also fearing that use of the new instrument might result in litigation from applicants who were rejected by admissions committees. The project has been shelved and shifted to the third area envisioned by the original MCAAP, that of establishing clinical performance criteria for medical students in the early clinical years.

Meanwhile, some interesting work in assessing the personality types of medical students is proceeding in some 18 medical schools (1977) as a result of extensive research in the use of the MBTI. Psychologist Mary McCaulley has been using the MBTI for more than 20 years on medical students and has found it a useful instrument in correlating personality types with the type of medical practice eventually chosen. Over the years, however, she has noted a change from the early 1950s when all 16 personality types defined by this instrument showed a fairly equal distribution, to the early 1970s when four of these "types" were conspicuously reduced. Interestingly, these four were the types most apt to favor office-based primary care careers—those which appear to be in shortest supply today. Furthermore, the scientifically oriented types were now markedly overrepresented and these had a strong predilection for specialization and/or an academic career.

McCaulley feels that this shift is probably a reflection of the medical school admission process *which tends to screen out those types which make the best primary care physicians*. These "sensing and feeling" types, as they have been called, simply don't do as well in test-taking or in the basic science areas but have a real feeling for people, communicate well, and do much better once they get into the clinical years; sometimes outperforming the "academic" types. If there is a real shortage of primary care physicians that continues into the future, Doctor McCaulley feels that medical schools will have to take a large part of the blame.[10]

The importance of the MBTI is heightened by the fact that the MCAAP had asked Doctor McCaulley to participate in their original noncognitive project before this was shelved for lack of funding. Fortunately, the American Medical Student Association Foundation is continuing to fund McCaulley's studies; it is ironical but commendable that the students are doing for themselves what the medical schools should have been providing. Unfortunately, medical schools and funding agencies must be wary and defensive when trying to improve selection methods in view of the current student and minority rights atmosphere. It is painful to reflect that some rejected applicants may be harming the chances of more qualified applicants because of lawsuits or other adverse action against the same medical schools which are trying to improve the selection and admission process. The applicants must recognize that they themselves, as well as the medical schools, have ethical obligations and that they too have a vital interest in seeing the selection process improved.

Although there has been some increased agitation for the acceptance of more applicants trained in the humanities, I am unaware of any hard evidence that humanistic students will be more humanitarian physicians than students without a strong background in the humanities. A humanist is not necessarily humanitarian; after all, one may fairly consider Machiavelli, Hitler, and Alexander the Great to have been humanists. I am also unaware of any evidence that so-called scientific or academic type physicians are any less humane than their "sensing-feeling" comrades. Both these points have undoubtedly annoyed some readers, but I promise to return to these allegations later.

Since we have a maldistribution, if not a shortage, of physicians both in terms of location and type of practice and specialty, it seems fair to ask whether applicants for medical school should not be considered partly on the basis of where they are likely to practice and whether or not they will do primary care. There is some evidence for the value of certain predictors of where an applicant is most likely to practice, at least in terms of urban or rural areas. And, as noted earlier, the MBTI can predict which types are most likely to enter primary or highly specialized care. But we immediately run into the problem of "equal protection under the law" clauses in the federal and some state constitutions which could view such selection as discriminatory. This is a swampy area in which there seems no clear trail, since both federal and state governments are currently seeking ways to induce physicians to locate in underserved locations. In addition, there are many officials in medical schools who say it is none of their concern as to where their graduates practice. This is a pressing ethical issue for medical schools and legislators to tackle, that is, the medical care needs of society as it relates to admissions policies.

The problems associated with the admission of minority applicants are even more potentially explosive. The federal government has been urging medical schools to accept more minority applicants. However, minority admission programs have run afoul of the equal protection clauses of both federal and state constitutions for at least two reasons: many students have been admitted under what amounts to a quota system and their academic records and assessment scores are generally lower than those of white applicants. Such preferential treatment has led to lawsuits from whites charging "reverse discrimination" in a curious twist of the equal protection clauses which were originally aimed at protecting blacks and other minorities. The most celebrated of these lawsuits to date is the Bakke case which ultimately went to the U. S. Supreme Court. In 1978 the high court rendered what has been called a "statesman-like" and "Solomonic" decision in this case which stated that while higher educational institutions could consider race as one preferential factor in the student selection process, they could not use a rigid quota system for such preference.[11] While it may take many years to establish firm legal guidelines for schools to follow, it is clearly established now that an applicant's background may be considered in the admission process.

Several points need to be made about minority admission programs. There is no question that many minority applicants are disadvantaged and have suffered many injustices, including inferior public education, and therefore *some* accommodations should be made. The increasing number of all applicants since World War II has steadily pushed up the MCAT and GPA averages, and yet no one is suggesting that the medical students accepted in the 1950s, for example, made inferior physicians.[12] Yet, the averages for students of that era are roughly equal to what minority applicants score today, making them comparable to applicants who are now physicians. If minority applicants could be selected on the basis of valid personality assessments as well as their academic aptitude, then we might have at least equally desirable medical students in terms of qualities like altruism, for example, and they may be more likely to enter primary care in underserved areas. Yet allowing minority students to enter medical school with lesser academic abilities than their white peers does them a disservice and harms the profession. Many minority students thus admitted have had to drop out later or repeat one or more training years. Once admitted, there is no chance for further preferential treatment, and ultimately there is the hurdle of licensure examinations which are the same for all candidates. Special remedial classes in medical schools have not worked out well, and there is a growing sentiment, realistically based, that needed remedial work be completed *prior* to entering medical school.

Qualified minority applicants with academic scores equal to those of an earlier generation make able physicians. However, there has been some agitation for the preferential selection of minority applicants with the mistaken idea that they will locate in ghetto or other medically underserved areas. This has not been the experience: these minority physicians too often select urban or suburban areas with a high income level as do many physicians, a phenomenon both understandable and regrettable. Some other means must be sought to attract new physicians to under-served areas.

Medical schools should continue to have the freedom to admit whom they wish to the study of medicine, but with this freedom must come the awesome responsibility of choosing well, in the light of their charters and the medical needs of society. In other words, medical schools must have the same combination of autonomy and responsibility that society has traditionally assigned to the individual professional person. Medical schools should not be compelled to select candidates solely on the basis of their test scores nor on their ethnic origin. The U.S. Supreme Court has made it clear that the race of an applicant may be considered but should not be the sole factor in making the selection. There is an urgent need for improved assessment methods for applicants, particularly in the area of personality characteristics and it is truly tragic that so little progress has been made in this area. Medical schools must feel free to utilize all reasonable screening methods for selecting the best candidates with immunity from lawsuits.

Meanwhile, we need more programs like those offered by several medical schools for minority students at the high school or college level designed to interest them in becoming doctors. These programs are usually given in the summer and offer selected and promising students an opportunity to see what medicine is all about. Visits are arranged to hospitals and clinics, private doctors' offices, and clinical laboratories and intensive instruction is given in the technique of test-taking, review of typical MCAT examinations, review of basic science material, and other areas. Positive programs like these make more sense than continuing to make accommodations at the admission level. Hopefully, the trend for such preferential treatment will ultimately disappear.

It seems at least questionable whether medical schools are getting the best all-around candidates they could because of overdependence on the applicant's academic abilities and too little knowledge about his/her personality. The relative importance of a scientific versus a humanities background is far from settled.

There is probably an optimal mix of characteristics among those students described by the MBTI as "sensing-feeling" and "academic" which is currently not represented in the medical schools. It seems reasonably clear that certain identifiable types of applicants make better primary care physicians and choose this field most often, a fact admissions committees ought to consider. These are also predictors for where an applicant will ultimately locate in terms of urban or rural areas. In addition to the academic and scientific evaluations, medical schools should push for better personality assessment instruments while using those now available. This is equally true in the case of minority students who could be chosen on a much broader selection base and would eliminate the policy of preferential selection that is so unsuccessful. *The key to getting better physicians in the categories and locations most needed by society is in an improved selection process.*

Let me here acknowledge the enormous amount of hard work and little thanks that is the lot of admissions committees everywhere. I served on such a committee for some time and although it taught me a lot about the admission jungle, there were times when we felt that this was one of the least appreciated jobs in the field of medicine. It may help them to realize that someone cares after all.

AFFECTIVE LEARNING IN MEDICAL SCHOOL

I have described earlier how a typical applicant is selected for medical school and some of the critical experiences he or she has had during the formal curriculum years. I propose now to reexamine the medical school years from two perspectives which in reality cannot be separated; one is what might be taught about the human side of medicine and the second is the special stresses and crisis points which face each student.

Two major points must be made first: Many medical educators feel that passage through the stress situations alone and unaided is necessary for medical students; a sort of rites of professional puberty. The second point is that all learning has affective as well as cognitive components, and hence the student will be shaped in both spheres by every learning experience. Medical students learn many of their roles by observing how their instructors, as role models, act toward patients and other members of the health-care community. In addition, the attitude of the faculty toward the students is an equally important factor for the growth and development of the nascent professional personality.

In the past several years a serious question has arisen over the desirability of requiring or even allowing the medical student to face these stress areas alone. Chase Kimball is a psychiatrist who for several years has been researching the effects of medical education on students. He has formed the interesting hypothesis that the medical education process has the potential of providing a greater humanization of the student than "any other experience afforded to mankind." [13] I stress "potential" because of the long-standing charge that medical education is a rather dehumanizing process as perceived by students and professional observers. Kimball and others have identified several "nodal points" during the medical curriculum that are regarded as especially stressful but that may offer equally great opportunity for humanization of the student. *The major factor which determines the humanization or dehumanization may be the philia demonstrated by the faculty toward the student in periods of stress.*

For example, the first nodal point is commonly the student's first encounter with a cadaver in anatomy class. Within a short time of entering medical school the student is expected to pick up a knife and begin to dissect a human body despite the fears and inhibitions about death in our culture. The way this is customarily handled is for the student to swallow his fears, make a show of bravado by coarse humor, and tell no one about his fears or bad dreams. An opportunity for enrichment or humanization is thus not only lost, but by denying the positive affectual aspects of such an encounter the student may become less feeling or more cynical. How different this might be if the student were given an opportunity to discuss this problem. For example, a selected number of faculty persons could provide a support system to work with students at this point, perhaps a humanist, a physician, a psychologist, and clergyman should be involved. Dissection of the human body could be discussed from the historical, religious, and psychologic aspects, but most importantly, the students could air their feelings and expand their affects. Equally important, the *student* will have been treated humanely.

There probably are unlimited opportunities for such humanizing or dehumanizing experiences in the medical education process, but perhaps a few more could be mentioned. The first contact with a dying patient, especially a younger one, can be quite traumatic. The first realization that medicine cannot always cure is stressful. The medical student has many worries, among them are the choice of practice, the knowledge he can never learn all of the material that he feels he should, and a fear of failure. He must remain in a psychosocial and economic holding pattern for several more years in what has been called "extended adolescence." The early didactic years of medical school are difficult; although the medical student is now a graduate student, he is not treated like one. His social security number is his identification; he may see no patients for several months and often lacks a physician role model. From his point of view, he has regressed, and although most students endure these early years, they undoubtedly lose many opportunities for affective learning and general enrichment.

Many schools have initiated reforms designed to overcome some of these problems. Such reforms include an early introduction to patient care, correlation of basic science work with actual patient contacts, and instruction for improving communication skills with patients. Many medical students have suggested helpful ways in which the curriculum can be improved, and they have also requested improved student counseling.[14] However, these innovations are not as common as one might wish and much remains to be done in these directions.

Medical students, like all college students, are provided with health-care services through the institutions in which they are enrolled. These services are often of an inferior and uncaring nature, a condition which does violence to a goal of training humane and compassionate physicians. This should concern all educators but especially those in medical schools. Medical students have many other vulnerabilities and there is a burning ethical responsibility here for medical schools which is not fully met.[15]

While going through these training years as an extended adolescent the typical student finds that the choice of medical specialty and what teaching hospital to select for residency training after graduation is very difficult. Preoccupation with such matters may adversely affect the student's performance and learning. Counseling by experienced personnel provided by the medical school would be extremely helpful to students who have asked for help in making these difficult decisions. Continued research with the MBTI or similar devices for helping students to choose seems indicated. It should not be assumed that these stresses cease with graduation from medical school; the typical resident works very hard, has heavy responsibilities, and may have second thoughts about his choice of specialty. In these postgraduate years the resident physician should also have easy access to capable personnel for counseling. In addition to the humane aspects of such support, it's good preventive medicine.

The Eastern Virginia Medical School has innovated some effective measures to help the humanizing experience of medical school. Their Human Values in Medicine program, headed by Doctor Donnie Self, holds a three day faculty-student retreat twice a year where topics of joint interest are discussed. Faculty and students get to know and care for one another as human beings. In addition to directing these retreats, the Human Values program makes many other contacts with students in the field of medical ethics and counseling services. Both faculty and students have been enthusiastic about these efforts and the school is building a reputation for attracting and reinforcing humane students.

In reading over the literature and in recalling my own student days, I am struck over and over by the sense of isolation and loneliness experienced by many medical students. Many find a sense of belonging and identity hard to come by and often long to share their feelings with classmates or faculty, but too few feel free to do so. As suggested earlier, students who are given humane and empathetic support by the faculty should be able to relate much better with their patients. If medical schools are selectively admitting the academic and competitive types described by McCaulley, these types often find it more difficult to relate warmly with patients; a difficulty compounded by a lack of sympathetic support to them during their medical school years.

Such a combination may well produce a maladjusted physician with continual problems in his or her practice years from failure to relate with patients or colleagues as human beings.

THE CURRICULUM MUDDLE

Prior to World War II the medical curriculum was highly conventional and standardized, with few if any electives, and students went through it largely unquestioning in lock-step fashion. This situation had been caused to a large degree by the post-Flexner push to crowd as much medical and clinical science as possible into the school years and by the impact of the knowledge explosion; educators felt there was little free time for electives or other innovations. Students felt similarly.

In the post-World War II period there were gradually increasing pressures from some students and faculty for more involvement in the social aspects of medicine plus more "relevant" topics and content in medical education. This agitation and turmoil reached its peak in the late 1960s and paralleled the countrywide revolutionary spirit of students in general. Some medical students wanted early patient contact, others wanted to set up and run free clinics for the poor in ghetto areas, while others wanted courses in human values, ethics, and the social sciences. With others, it was hard to tell what they wanted; it was almost rebellion for rebellion's sake.

Underneath all of this activity for reform there was some consensus among medical educators and students that medical schools should offer more contact in the "soft sciences," the human values area, and nonmedical enrichment courses in general. This is somewhat paradoxical because student cynicism often seems to be directed at courses seen as *not* purely "medical." Such cynicism may be justified in schools where such courses are perceived as merely token and where few of the principles that are taught are practiced. Although the agitation for reform did lead to some positive curriculum changes, these were not widespread enough, and this has undoubtedly caused more cynicism.

As early as 1961 the AMA recommended that each medical school develop and present a *required* course "in ethics and socio-economic principles" and that medical schools cooperate with state licensing boards and medical associations to insure that students become acquainted with "practical problems of ethics and socio-economic principles and their proper solutions." These recommendations had very little direct impact on the medical schools insofar as implementation was concerned. If the AMA had been able to award funds to schools desiring to initiate or expand the recommended programs, it might have helped, but unfortunately, the AMA did not dispense, it only prescribed.

In an effort to find out what was going on in this area of teaching, I conducted a survey of U.S. and Canadian medical schools in 1966 and found that some 40 percent of the schools which responded to the questionaire indicated they were offering some instruction or contact in medical ethics or religion in medicine and which, for lack of a better name, I called "ethico-religious" instruction.[16] Some of this contact or instruction was minimal, for example, a clergyman may have participated in some of the teaching conferences as the only manifestation of religion in medicine. I also learned that some medical educators were opposed to the teaching of human values and stated that values could not be "taught"; it had to be visible in faculty and staff attitudes throughout the entire curriculum. If the recommendations of the AMA had not fallen on totally deaf ears, they certainly encountered many with hearing problems.

In 1966, with the support of the Department of Religion of George Washington University, I initiated an elective course for second-year medical students at the same university under the title, "Medicine, Religion, and Healing" (MRH). The course was offered for one semester for one hour per week and dealt with the religious values of the patient, the place of religion in healing, the rights of the patient, the tradition of the professional person, and a team approach to healing which included a clergyman, and the concept of total care for the totality of man. The content of the course was subsequently expanded to include many more medical ethical issues.[17]

The first course was felt to be quite successful, judging from the number and reactions of the students who elected it, but in succeeding years the course suffered from the competitive effects of a growing number of "hard medicine" electives for second-year students. We were to learn that courses of this kind waxed and waned in popularity for many unknown reasons but that support from both students and faculty was essential. Positive faculty support was most helpful while passive go-ahead-and-do-your-thing attitudes were viewed as negative by the students. Merely permitting a course like this was not enough; students had to perceive active endorsement by the faculty. Some faculty attended the sessions, and this was viewed as positive support.

More important things needed to be discovered; for instance, were such courses effective in making students more humane? Based on some questionnaire surveys (which are notoriously unreliable) of medical students, I was prepared to believe the MRH course was useful in changing their attitudes toward being more empathetic and humanitarian.[18] However, despite such wishful thinking, I concluded that more objective methods for assessing the effects of such a course were needed. In succeeding years two different groups were assessed as to certain precourse and postcourse values, using an appropriate psychological test. The results were far from conclusive, and there were defects in the methods I used. However, the results did suggest that the course might be of value in retarding the expected erosion of values or the increasing cynicism normally displayed by medical students during the medical school years.[19] It was equally possible that courses of this type were most often selected by those students who were already more empathetic and humane and such students might be more resistant to a loss of values.

Are compassion and empathy matters that can be taught? Can one teach medical ethics? Those who have had experience in offering courses similar to mine are generally agreed that you can't "teach" such qualities and topics in the literal sense. Furthermore, the power of the professionalization process to change certain basic attitudes is much less than has been supposed. However, I agree with Louis Lasagna, who says that offering such courses does have value in sensitizing students to important ethical issues and in suggesting ways to deal with them while reinforcing previously held values in this area.[20] Lasagna also suggests that a single course is simply inadequate for an optimal exposure of students to ethical issues and the need for humaneness; these matters must be continually reemphasized and reinforced by practice and precept throughout the professional life of the physician.

In a related study of medical educators, Babbie concluded that good people simply make good doctors and what most of us might agree constitutes "goodness" is determined long before admission to medical school. For example, a medical school might be able to sway a student into selecting family practice rather than the surgical career originally selected, but there would be little influence on the manner in which that practice was conducted. As a logical sequel to these conclusions, he felt that "more enlightened recruiting" of medical students was needed to help produce better physicians. As examples, Babbie showed that attitudes of medical faculty members toward socialized medicine and the right to die were the product of social beliefs rather than medical training. Furthermore, such factors as age, religious background, geographic area of rearing, and political beliefs were strong determinants of attitudes toward such medical-social issues.[21]

Babbie also concluded that more scientific physicians were not less humane than the less scientific; in fact, more scientifically oriented physicians were more likely to accept the findings of the behavioral and social sciences which have a deterministic view of man. Thus the poor, for example, are not poor of their own choosing but because of forces beyond their control which have been demonstrated by economists and social scientists.

Babbie's findings and conclusions, along with those of others, have implications for teaching as well as the selection process. Since "medical" attitudes toward certain ethical issues (abortion, right to die, for example) are really based on one's social and religious beliefs, it would seem wise to discuss such issues directly in terms of their social or religious natures rather than as disguised medical problems. Helping students to understand some of the determinants responsible for certain of their attitudes could promote an open atmosphere for discussion and retard the formation of cynicism. Physicians who understand the basis for some of their feelings should be able to understand their patients better and communicate more effectively.

Should courses dealing with these subjects be required? I have mixed feelings in this regard since some students who are indifferent or hostile to such concepts may be alienated or further alienated by being required to take such courses. However, course material dealing with ethics, religion, social issues, and other topics that may create negativism can be blended into a continuing course that deals with more neutral items, such as medical economics or jurisprudence. Such a tactic might avoid making controversial subject matter conspicuous—a risk that one runs by setting a course off by itself. My closing thought is that in a risk-benefit sense, it is probably better to expose all students to vital matters such as ethics and human values at the risk of alienating a few.

How should such material be presented? As stated above, it should be part of a continuing core program devoted to the human side of medicine. The subject matter and instructors should not be isolated so that they appear to be an adjunct to medicine rather than a part of the mainstream. It is important to have physicians participate in the course work, but allied health professionals should also be used as much as possible since the students need to realize that the complexities of modern health care require the help of many disciplines.

Various formats are possible. For example, there may be lectures with discussions following, or groups of students may be assigned topics for discussion which they then research and present with discussion afterward. The case-study method makes the course more relevant to medicine, and a new book of case studies in medical ethics by Robert M. Veatch is now available.[22] Videotapes, films, and casettes are useful and available. Individual students may use materials for self-instruction at the learning resources center which is a part of every modern medical school. For home study or individual use there is the very useful book by Howard Brody, *Ethical Decision in Medicine*, a self-instructional text which takes the student through many case studies and allows him to make ethical decisions and shows some alternative choices.[23] This book represents a remarkable achievement since Brody wrote it as an undergraduate medical student, and it fills a definite gap in medical ethics teaching.

What should be the content of a medical ethics program? This is absolutely open-ended for the reason that bears repeating: medical ethics is the right conduct of medical practice. Ethical material should be interwoven into a core course that deals with other aspects of human medicine such as social medicine and medical economics. Any of the material presented in this book could be used in such a core course. Above all, presentations must be contemporary, relevant, and credible. They also should be presented with the same academic rigor as any recognized "medical" course, or many students will perceive them as less important as well as "non-medical."

The number of medical schools that offer some exposure to medical ethics has increased greatly in the decade since my 1966 survey. Veatch and Sollitto conducted a similar survey of medical schools in the U.S. in 1974 and found that 97 of 107 schools reporting indicated some kind of medical ethics teaching with 56 of them conducting conferences, lectures, or seminars in this area.[24] It would be a rare medical school today which offered no teaching in medical ethics. This enormous increase since my 1966 survey should represent a genuine response to both societal and student needs, but there is always an element of me-tooism in educational circles. Success spurs imitation. Popularity is one possible component of this success in the teaching of ethics, but the real test is how well ethical principles are incorporated into all aspects of medical teaching—including the admissions and selection process.

Paralleling the rise of interest in medical ethics is a renewed interest in the study of the humanities in the premedical curricula or even in medical school.[25] I say "renewed" because the same view was expressed nearly a century ago by the noted medical educator William Osler who stated that the physician should have the "education of a gentleman if not of a scholar."[26] Some medical schools now require a year of behavioral science or other humanities in the premedical years in addition to certain science courses.

Probably no medical educator in this country believes more strongly in the value of humanistic studies for medical students than Edmund Pellegrino. In the preface of his book *Humanism and the Physician*, he writes about the value of a "humanistic medical education" for producing "competent, considerate, and conversant physicians" and further states:

> The humanities have a unique place in this effort. They sensitize to values, they inculcate the liberal arts as attitudes of mind, and they prepare physicians for a life of satisfaction as well as competence....
>
> The move among so many medical schools to teach the humanities, and to examine values, promises to be the most important innovation in medical education in the next quarter century.[27]

Doctor Pellegrino is a humanist by virtue of his education and a humanitarian physician. However, this happy combination of qualities does not prove cause and effect as he sincerely believes. At the very most enrichment courses or studies like these (including ethics) have only retarded the normal development of cynicism in some medical students as was mentioned earlier. Furthermore, there is some evidence that such teaching efforts may increase cynicism for reasons I discussed earlier. Certainly a knowledge of the humanities is helpful in developing a personal orientation in general and medical ethics and for understanding the human condition. There is, furthermore, some public expectation that the physician be a cultured person and have the "education of a gentleman," an expectation that is not always fulfilled. But possession of all these qualities, desirable though they may be, does not alone make one more humanitarian. A broad education ought to make a good physician a better one, but there are no guarantees.

At the same time the necessity of an undergraduate background in natural science for a physician may be seriously doubted. In a recent study four investigators from a medical school have concluded that medical students from natural science and nonscience undergraduate backgrounds did not differ significantly in their grades in the first two years of medical school, nor in their clinical performance in the third year, nor in their scores on parts I and II of the National Board Medical Examination. Choice of type of residency among graduating seniors was also independent of their undergraduate majors.[28] This study adds substantial weight to the argument for a broad undergraduate background if we really want more widely cultured physicians, but the authors make it clear that their study does not deal with the need for scientific *aptitude* in medical students.

For reasons that I hope may now be clearer, I have little faith in the ability of medical school curricula to improve the basic personality of a student and, if such be the case, it constitutes a strong argument for a better selection of students who already possess those personal qualities which are determined to be desirable. Medical schools have an equal ethical obligation to carefully select their faculty on the basis of their personal qualities as well as their expertise.

SOME CONCLUDING THOUGHTS

I stated earlier that the influence of the medical school years on the basic attitudes and belief systems of students was much less than had previously been supposed, and courses in medical ethics or the humanities, for example, would not change a Machiavelli into a St. Francis. However, there is evidence for the value of such enrichment programs in reinforcing certain views and values held by some students which appear to be necessary (or at least helpful) in the making of a good physician. There may be some additional value in introducing certain ethical concepts and values to students previously unaware of them, with the hope that some students would be sensitized to certain important areas, even if their values are not changed in medical school. Then too, it is conceivable that some of the "cutthroat premeds" might ultimately come to a more humane world view some time after graduation from medical school. Like Pellegrino, I want to believe that enrichment studies would transform all medical students, but I know better.

The outlook is far from pessimistic despite my negative findings and conclusions. I have also indicated some positive conclusions such as the great importance of admitting the best candidates to medical school with a balance of academic-intuitive and sensing-feeling types. If we want more humane doctors of medicine, we must recruit humane students and humane faculty to interact together. The complexity of medical practice today also demands some exposure of the medical student to medical economics and medical social issues. Mere courses in ethics and the humanities or other enrichment courses are simply inadequate. If goodness can be taught, as Socrates maintained, then it must be taught early in life and not be taken on as a remodeling job in medical school.

At this point I propose to sketch out some of the features that I think most important to incorporate in a medical school curriculum, recognizing that many of them are already being tried in several schools. I shall assume that an optimally balanced mix of both "feeling" and "academic" type students has been admitted. These students will have had a minimum personality assessment by instruments such as the Meyer-Briggs Type Indicator and the Minneapolis Multiphasic Personality Inventory. The first few days of school would be spent in small group discussions between students and faculty advisors and counselors, getting acquainted with one another and learning what to expect in the first few weeks and months. Since human anatomy is normally the first major course, a select "support committee" would be formed to tell students what to expect in regard to the dissection of a cadaver and to allow students an opportunity to vent their anxieties. Periodic sessions would be held with different small groups during the first several weeks.

Each student should be assigned to a physician faculty advisor after first-year registration and be required to make a certain number of contacts with the advisor during the year. This requirement is important because many students feel that they are not supposed to voice complaints or problems. Such an attitude is tied in with the traditional but useless notion that a student must sink or swim on his own in those first difficult months. In addition to being an empathetic listener, the advisor would serve as a physician role model for the student which is sorely needed in the basic science years when patients and physicians are rarely seen. Either the advisor or the student should feel free to dissolve the relationship if it is unsatisfactory and seek another liason.

It is most important to new medical students to feel that there is at least one physician with whom they can relate. This relationship can be utilized in other ways; for example, during the concentration in basic medical science it is very helpful to have a physician-coordinator point to the connection between these science courses and the world of medicine. Thus, the student in biochemistry would be taken to the bedside or clinic to see a patient with biochemical lesions such as are present in diabetes, kidney failure, liver disease, and so on.

First year students are often assigned to emergency rooms or physicians' offices as observers so that they will have early contact with clinical medicine. While some of these contacts are well received many students tire quickly of this observor role when they discover there is little they can do for patients at this point and other more pressing priorities confront them. Such an experience should be offered with no penalty for dropping out. Some schools have assigned first-year students to families which they follow throughout the medical school years. Another approach has been to assign a student to a pregnant woman who is then followed through the delivery and early child-rearing process. Students should be asked to make home visits on selected patients whom they have seen in the clinics or hospital to note the home conditions and other environmental factors. Efforts such as these intended to give some insight into community medicine and family dynamics have been well-received.[29]

There are many studies which support the notion that patients perceive the empathy or humanitarianism of a physician by the manner in which the medical encounter is conducted, in other words, the interviewing skills of the physician are all-important. It is possible to train medical students to increase these skills and to increase their degree of empathy in the doctor-patient relationship.[30] Therefore, some training of this type should be included in the ideal curriculum and is now required at a few schools.

Social medicine and related ethical issues form one of the most neglected areas in medical education, a point graphically made by Doctor John H. Knowles when he told a Senate subcommittee that the AAMC had been as conservative and backward as the AMA in this regard. He added that these two major political forces of American medicine "have stuck their heads in the sand and put their backsides to the socio-economic problems of medicine."[31] In the decade since that observation, too few medical schools have responded to the unmet teaching needs in the area of social medicine.

The subject matter of social medicine is almost limitless since it concerns the health and well-being of society and the study of areas where health and health care are deficient and what can be done to improve them. Some of the issues related to social medicine are health care as a right, health-care provision for those unable to afford it, preventive medicine and public-health measures, barriers to health care, self-health care, and health-care education. Other concerns of social medicine are the roles that poverty, ignorance, and the environment play in the causation of disease, social injustice, exploitation of patients by health-care providers, inequalities of health care, medically underserved areas, number of primary care physicians as compared with those in secondary and tertiary care, overutilization of hospitals, abuses in nursng homes, fraud and abuse of medical services covered by third-party carriers, and consumer participation in the management of health-care facilities; to name but a few. Social medicine seeks ways to improve the health of society at all levels but especially for those, like the poor, who do not enjoy the better health status of the more affluent.Medical students need exposure to all of these topics.

In their formal school years medical students should learn not only the basics of running a private medical office but also such things as cost containment, optimal use of hospitals, economic advantages of various medical insurance and other health care plans, the economics of proposed national health-care plans, a comparison of fee-for-service with a salaried basis of practice, the faults of Medicaid-Medicare, and why some 40 million Americans lack adequate health coverage. There are some signs of progress in these areas.[32]

Instruction should also be presented in medical history, important features of religious belief in a medical context, medical sociology, how to deal with loss and grief, the dying patient, roles of other health care professionals, and humanities as they relate to medicine. With tongue in cheek I might also suggest that any time left over be used to study clinical medicine! To be totally serious, it is entirely possible to cover all of these topics and have adequate time for the learning of clinical medicine as well; whether an adequate balance of human and scientific medicine will be offered, depends on the mentality of the individual medical school. The more the human side of medicine is integrated into clinical or scientific medicine, the better will be the teaching of holistic medicine. Ideally, the human aspects of medicine should be covered while the student is working with patients. Since this may be inconvenient, a continuing core course can at least survey the field of human medicine along the lines of the topics and areas suggested. It should be possible in any clinical presentation to bring out the human as well as the scientific aspects of the case. "Poverty" is just as important an entry on the patient's problem list as "bronchial asthma."

Those who feel that there is simply not enough time to teach the elements of medicine in four years let alone the human aspects might consider what Kelly West has called the seven futilities of medical education:

1. Only a small portion of the current body of medical knowledge can be taught in four years.
2. Much of the knowledge which will be employed in the student's future career is not known today and therefore cannot be taught.
3. Not all that is taught is learned.
4. A small part of what is taught is erroneous.
5. A portion of what is learned will soon be obsolete.
6. The physicians of the future (including family physicians) will be specialists, and so some of what they learn will have limited relevance to their future careers.
7. Of that which is taught and learned and relevant, much is quickly forgotten.[33]

Perhaps educators should worry less about cramming in so much clinical medicine and devote more time to the human side of the art. Keeping West's aphorisms in mind might help medical educators retain a little balance in the presentation of the art and science of medicine.

There has been a curious lack of critical examination by the medical schools in regard to their own corporate ethics. They must be bound by the same ethics as individual physicians, with responsibilities to students and society. As corporate stewards, our medical schools must carefully nurture that which they have been given in trust and know that there will be a time of accounting for their stewardship. The medical education community should join forces and push research in the selection methods of students with the same avidity with which they push medical research. They should seek ways to improve the present disparate efforts to make students more humane. Since medical schools use public funds, they have a contractual and ethical obligation to help place their graduates where they are needed, balancing individual and societal rights. Finally, if at any pont in the education process a student should be judged less than adequate for a career in medicine, then he or she must be rehabilitated or dropped from the program; this responsibility has not been met as it should be.

In the village life of many eastern Mediterranean countries, the teacher is the most revered figure because of a centuries-old tradition of respect for wisdom and knowledge. Not just knowledge, but wisdom and knowledge. Wisdom cannot be taught but it is essential for enlightened teaching.

CHAPTER 13

TOWARD AN ORDERED WHOLE

We live in a world of twisted and tangled values. We currently champion human rights, but two decades ago at least part of the United States was still practicing the principles of segregation. We punished Axis "war criminals" at Nuremberg after World War II, but in the same conflict we dropped two nuclear bombs that destroyed two Japanese cities and some two hundred thousand human beings, most of them civilians. We pursued a senseless and brutal war in Indochina, but we have trouble at home adopting a sound policy for therapeutic abortion or euthanasia. We decry the fact that more than half the world population lacks enough food while the amount we spend on pet food would probably feed most of the hungry. We had unrelieved urban blight and violence in the ghettos while NASA was spending billions on space exploration.

These value coflicts are not unique to the U.S. nor are they a product of our age: they have existed in all times and cultures. Man does not appear to have a propensity for clear and consistent thinking. It has often seemed easier to fight than to reason or to destroy in the name of love or religion. In such a light it is hard to understand how the tradition of medical ethics has continued to develop and survive in the presence of so many hostile forces. Apparently the subject has attracted enough good and thinking people out of each generation to make its survival possible.

The practice of ethical medicine within the context of my interpretation is to help another human in need for altruistic reasons, in other words, in the service-first tradition. This act or impulse to help another seems very ancient and is generally approved by various cultures. Basically, we all need to feel love and concern at times, and a tradition which calls for service and responsibility in the care of humans is commonly viewed as reflecting that kind of loving concern. Thinking people can see that the right conduct of medical practice requires using the entire body of ethical tradition which I refer to as the "Hippocratic legacy." Although this body of medical ethics has slowly developed over thousands of years, so far as we know, there has always been medicine's self-imposed ethical demand that a physician be a person of purity, who cares for others and strives to be competent. That is the core of the Hippocratic legacy or whatever we choose to call it, a tradition that endures because some physicians down through the ages have felt it to be right.

I say "some physicians" because it is obvious that the medical community suffers from the same confusion and value conflicts that trouble society generally, and it is equally obvious that medical ethics are no more practiced in this last quarter of the twentieth century than are ethics in society at large. So what could there possibly be about ethical behavior that makes some of us feel right about it and impels some of us to follow ethical conduct and induce others to do the same? Could this be some kind of instinctive or intuitive behavior? Or is there some unknown force or law of nature for right conduct to which we imperfectly respond? Could it be both or neither?

To respond to these questions, we might begin by taking a fresh look at the cosmos and the world around us.[1] There appears to be a general state of order in the universe which is constantly reaffirmed by scientific observation and inductive reasoning. Galaxies, stars, and planets all move with predictive regularity and harmony. Within this planet of ours there appears to be a subset of the universal order; a biosphere or ecosystem containing a remarkable number of life forms nicely balanced with each other and living in reasonable harmony. Within the harmonious milieu of this biosphere, man lives and moves and has his being.

An ancient recognition of this universal and worldly order probably initiated the concept that is known as natural law.

There are several meanings for this term: for example, there is natural law which regulates all of the universe but I shall be using the term in a more restricted sense. My definition says there exists certain precepts, or norms, or rules, of good and right conduct which are discoverable by man, which he is required to follow, and which are a part of the larger, universal natural law. Assuming that there is a natural law for the conduct of mankind, it is possible for us to follow this natural law and be in harmony with it or fail to follow it and be in disharmony. It is known that in primitive cultures man sees himself as being at one with nature and lives in harmony with it. By the time of Hippocrates the Greeks had developed the notion that the *physis* (the wholeness or constitution or nature of man) must be in harmony with the larger *physis*, that is, the natural world and natural law, and they reasoned that disease could result from a disruption of that harmony.[2]

Natural law was a cornerstone of Stoic philosophy, whose followers believed that the fundamental ethical principles that underlay the legal systems of all nations were reducible to the principles of natural law. The Stoics also believed that God was everywhere and in every human and that He settled and arranged everything. Stoicism was embraced by many Romans, including the noted orator, Cicero, who left us a classical definition of natural law: "True law is right reason in agreement with Nature; it is of universal application, unchanging, and everlasting ... there will be one master and one ruler, that is, God, over us all, for He is the author of this law, its promulgator, and the enforcing judge."[3] Thomas Aquinas, the greatest theologian of the medieval Christian Church, proclaimed similarly that natural law was of divine origin and pointed to the dignity and power of man, inasmuch as we are called to participate actively in the rational order of the universe because of our rational nature. Aquinas also emphasized that natural law provided the basis for ethics because of man's participation in the ordered scheme of things, that is, an obligation to follow natural law.[4]

But man can and does violate natural law and thus can be in disharmony with it which can result in disease or the unnatural condition noted in the Hippocratic writings and later by the

Romans.[5] Since 1552 the English Book of Common Prayer has contained a prayer which indicates that failure of right conduct, whether by commission or omission, would cause a lack of health. Paul Tillich has drawn attention to disease as a disruption of wholeness and reminds us that health or wholeness is identical to "salvation" as that word should be understood in the New Testament. This proper understanding means wholeness or health in all dimensions; mind, body, and spirit.[6] It appears that the concept of disease as related to a lack of harmony with or violation of natural law is a very old one.

The understanding or interpretation of natural law has changed somewhat over the centuries, but certain basic premises remain the same: natural law is part of the universal order, and men must seek to discover and follow these laws. In the post-Reformation era there was a gradual movement to emphasize the rights of man deriving from natural law, and this notion inspired much of the rhetoric and sentiment of the American and French revolutions in the eighteenth century. However, with the parallel rise of the age of science, natural law suffered a decline in the nineteenth century largely because it was not subject to the same type of proof that was used for natural sciences. Nonetheless, natural law has survived and has been given new life by some twentieth century writers like Jacques Maritain and C. S. Lewis.

Physicians, trained as scientists, tend to be wary and sceptical of new or unproven or "unscientific" theories and treatments. Natural law cannot be "proven" with mathematical precision as can the law of gravity. However, is it not possible that violation of natural law produces effects not immediately visible? We have seen that in the past many men have believed that disease could be one result of violating natural laws. Now physicians know that bacteria and viruses caused infectious disease. But what about the ruinous life-styles, for example, that some people follow? Couldn't these represent disharmony, and doesn't this predispose one to infection? What about the cultural malaise and boredom caused by affluence? Could it be that greed on the part of some, causing gross inequality in the distribution of the world's goods, is a violation of natural law? We may call such malaise a neurosis, but will that change the causal mechanics?

Many of us remember the balanced aquarium in introductory biology, where fish and plants lived together in a microcosm of harmony. The fish ate the plants and gave off nitrogenous waste and carbon dioxide which were needed by the plants; the plants gave off oxygen which the fish needed for life, and so on. Disruption of this harmony by cutting the cycle at any point causes death of all the life in the aquarium. The pollution of our earth's ecosystem, the biosphere, may not produce immediate harmful effects but what about the long-term ones? We know that overpopulation has some harmful effects, but do we know them all and what are we doing about it? "Papa Doc" was right; birth control was not needed where the quality of life was dismal, but now that it is so improved in much of the world, there must be a balancing check on the birth rate. What happens if we permanently disrupt one of our major ecological balances? Can we afford to find out the hard way? The answers to these rhetorical questions seem clear enough: we are not conforming as we should to the principles of natural law (which includes our Hippocratic legacy) which are necessary to save our world from almost certain destruction otherwise.

Van Rensselaer Potter, a well-regarded medical scientist, has popularized the word "bioethics" in his book by the same name.[7] Bioethics is the right conduct, the ethical conduct, that must exist between man and the global environment and is absolutely necessary for survival.[8] Human ethics may not be separated from our ecology; bioethics involves our entire biosphere and therefore, involves man just as it involves all other life forms. Our ethical conduct, in this larger view, must extend to our worldly environment (and beyond since the start of space exploration) as well as to other human beings. I consider Potter's Bioethical Creed important enough to include in the appendix because it spells out some essential beliefs we must follow if we are to be bioethical. Perhaps now the importance of the stewardship concept can be seen as more relevant: each person, by following the stewardship role, is placing himself in harmony with natural law by acting as conserver, protector, and manager of his lifetime gifts from the Creator.

More recently the discipline or movement known as sociobiology has hypothesized a scientific rationale for human behavior which would lend credibility to the natural law theory. C. H. Waddington is a respected geneticist who believes that ethical human behavior is the optimal conduct that humans can exercise toward one another and that the learning of ethical behavior is a necessary part of human evolution.[9] Furthermore, this is a continually developing process which requires both genetic and social transmission. Thus, there may be within humans a specific need for ethical learning which is genetically determined and is maximal in young children and is a time when there is optimal receptivity to ethical input. Ideally, at this time the child should receive ethical teaching from his elders, that is, the beliefs and practices which have been culturally transmitted from one generation to another through the ages. This "socio-genetic" theory is similar to the imprinting theory for the early learning by young animals or the sensitivity to stimuli displayed by a single cell and which we call feedback. It speaks to the importance of man as a social animal so that the distilled wisdom and experience of the ages can be passed on to each child. It also points to the fact that much early learning from one's elders is too variable and should be improved; this possibility could greatly alter our educational policies.

Other sociobiologists agree that much of human behavior is determined by our genetic makeup as well as social forces. For example, it has been postulated that genes are self-programmed to insure their own survival by the propogation of many diverse types. Thus, altruism or other ethical behavior may serve the function of protecting humans only for the purpose of protecting the genes, a hypothesis which has led to the term "selfish genes."[10] In a sense, the genes are immortal since they continue to duplicate themselves and survive through the medium of offspring and only the bodies which contain them for a short time are mortal.

In any case, a fundamental premise of sociobiology is that genes serve as regulators of the social actions of all animals, including man. There can be no doubt that genes ultimately modify behavior but to what extent in man remains to be determined.

It may well be that when man entered the age of civilization, he turned his back on his ethical stirrings or the socio-genetic mechanism for right conduct with which he had lived comfortably as a primitive. If so, the story of the fall of man would have a firm evolutionary basis and would represent allegorically the disharmony between man and the laws established by the Creator. It does not seem too remote a possiblity that ethical programming in humans is an integral part of the ordered world and universe. It appears likely that some human behavior is genetically determined, and that a portion is designed to protect and preserve humanity. If we assume that some human behavior is genetically programmed, the obvious corollary is: how may we develop our lost sensitivity to that programming?

It is tempting to speculate on the future role of genetic engineering in the area of human conduct. If, as some natural law philosophers believe, all men have been given intelligence so that they may be partners with the Creator in the management of their destiny and evolution, then genetic manipulation is integral to that scheme. The continuing cycle of life and death is in part required so that our genes may adapt to a changing environment or other stimuli, but such changes take thousands of years. However, genetic manipulation in the laboratory may make it possible to produce beneficial changes in our behavior and physical beings within the space of a generation and such man-induced changes can also be viewed as part of the natural order we were intended to fulfill.

Obviously, the greatest wisdom is required in any effort to control our evolution, but the rewards would be considerable. *The Henderson Monster* is the title of a recent television drama which portrayed a molecular geneticist almost devoid of ethics in his research into genetic manipulation or "recombinant DNA." His consuming lust for personal fame and recognition in his field overshadowed all other considerations. Such an attitude could, of course, lead to haste or sloppy technique in his work, and so the monster in the title was not some terrible genetic hybrid let loose upon the world but rather the unethical scientist who would make such an accident possible. The possibility of some disaster in this area will become as real as a nuclear holocaust is now. We have indeed entered an era that will test whether men can responsibly act as partners with the Creator; if ever our world needed wisdom it is now.

Some of this discussion is reminiscent of the arguments which were common in the early part of this century over the relative importance of heredity and environment in the determination of human intelligence. Insofar as human behavior is concerned, it would seem that both are needed and equally important. The scenario resembles an exposed photographic film: if the latent image (genetic programming) is present, then proper chemical development (ethical input) will bring it out, but if the latent image isn't there, no amount of developing will evoke it. In time it may be possible to genetically program a better image, but for now the best course is to seek ways to increase our sensitivity to the programming we now have but appear to be ignoring. Supported by this improved knowledge and acting within the context of *philia*, we must continue to struggle with the ethical problems which beset us. We have learned to modify our environment and our state of health to some degree. Only human beings are equipped to both break natural law and find ways to restore themselves to harmony with it.

In such a search for wholeness, natural law exponents would say that by exercising right conduct man can again be in conformity with natural law which would restore natural order and wholeness. Theology would hold that man must get right with God by recognizing and confessing his faults or sins, resolving to do better, and then could be brought to salvation. Natural science would demonstrate that a break in an ecosystem would throw an orderly system into disorder. When the break is restored, the system is sometimes restored to order and harmony. There is a definite unity in all three of these views.

Modern medical care has improved the health and longevity of man to only a limited degree because its usual approach is to treat disease as disease rather than by seeking out and removing root causes. More than a century ago a general trend began toward improved sanitation, a better living standard, and higher standards of purity for food, drugs, and water which did more to advance the health and longevity of Western man than did medical science.[11] In other words, correcting the root causes of some diseases resulted in more health improvement than did treating the diseases alone. Although we may like to think, scientifically speaking, that we had discovered the causes of specific human diseases, is it not possible that there is one ultimate disorder in man that is responsible for many other illnesses?

The basic disorder in man may be his failure to practice *philia* toward his fellow man. This imperative is stated as one of the two great commandments and comes out of the theological wisdom of the Old and New Testaments. It is one way of expressing a natural law. Failure to observe that law has resulted in disorder and harm to man and his environment. This lack of love ranges from simple neglect of another human being to exploitation, oppression, and destruction of others. This failure to exercise care and concern for our neighbors has caused the social illnesses of poverty, overpopulation, starvation, vice, crime, violence, pollution, warfare, and rape of our natural resources. These social disorders have directly and indirectly caused both somatic and mental disease in humans.

This lack of love for one another may be manifested in the neglect, exploitation, or oppression of others for one's own gain. Affluence from whatever source produces a surplus of leisure which often creates boredom. Boredom, in turn, causes a pursuit of pleasure with ever-diminishing returns which ultimately creates more boredom. We are currently witnessing the consequences of affluence: for those who have it, there are increasing rates of mental disease, suicide, rampant sexual aberration, alcoholism, and drug abuse—all symptoms of despair from failure to find contentment. For those who have it not, there is increased crime, increased mental disease, drug abuse, alcoholism, and suicide—from the same failure to find contentment! In addition, the poor have more chronic disease, a shorter life expectancy, and a higher infant mortality rate than the affluent.

There is a theory of natural rights which arises from natural law and is considered to date back to the Stoics.[12] Natural rights was prominent in the rhetoric of the American and French revolutions and predicates a natural equality among men. One may reason that we are all intended to share equally in the pleasures and material goods of this world and therefore some should not have an excessive portion of these material goods at the expense of others. Affluence for some may mean poverty for others; such inequalities in distribution of the goods of this world seems to be a violation of natural law in a community or global sense. All of the social ills of mankind could be viewed as human pollution resulting from a failure to care for one another:

But it is not only the pollutions and degradations of the atmosphere and the ocean that threaten the quality of life at the planetary level. There are threats, too, of disease spreading among undernourished children, of protein deficiency maiming the intelligence of millions, of spreading illiteracy combined with rising numbers of unemployed intellectuals, of landless workers streaming to the squalid cities, and worklessness growing there to engulf a quarter of the working force. An acceptable strategy for planet Earth must, then, explicitly take account of the fact that the natural resource most threatened with pollution, most exposed to degradation, most liable to irreversible damage is not this or that species, not this or that plant or biome or habitat, not even the free airs or the great oceans. It is man himself.[13]

An attack on human pollution will require the coordinated activities of all governments and many people. We must learn much from other professions, especially the social and behavioral sciences. Medicine is not only able to relieve, comfort, and heal disease but in the stewardship reference, via its preventive, educational, and conservationist aspects, can help to promote a better world. A physician who would be the good steward of health his traditions require must first inform himself and his peers about that tradition and its demands; a task too long neglected. The medical profession needs to recognize that health care must be expanded from a system of episodic care of specific illness into a truly comprehensive and preventive approach to include the social ills of mankind.

Medicine cannot hope to successfully treat specific disease in those who live in a state of despair or apathy that comes from being deprived or abused in various ways. These victims of social ills often have no motivation to get well. Lack of attention to this basic fact is one of the reasons social medical programs in the U.S. have not been more successful. Programs such as Medicaid-Medicare use a medical-care system which is basically disease-oriented and episodic in nature for the health-care needs of the poor and elderly, many of whom simply have no wish to get well. One has to believe that life is worth living before he or she makes the effort to continue, and it is clear that many people in this world lack that belief.

If the medical profession is to accept the challenge of participation in the attack on social ills, it must do two things. The first is to clean up the mess within its own house by instituting reforms in those areas which need it. Secondly, medicine must develop a social awareness and conscience so that social ills can be perceived and treatment effectively planned and executed. The single overriding need within the medical profession is the development of a pervasive ethical mentality within a context of brotherly love which will generate guidelines for conduct and responsiveness to human need.[14] One must be well himself before he can effectively treat another; an ethical mentality provides the hygiene needed by medicine to maintain its health. If physicians thoroughly support an attack on the social ills of mankind, in addition to practicing orthodox medicine, they will certainly be much more in harmony with natural law by using this comprehensive approach to total health.

Are these thoughts merely an ideal or a vision of a better world? If we are to work for a state in which man and the world lives in harmony, we must begin with that vision or ideal. Medicine is both art and science but not just an applied science: it is also a social science in which physicians must work with other disciplines to correct some of the basic social ills I have discussed and which are disruptions of natural law. We need to keep working for a better future while bearing in mind one fundamental maxim: we must love one another and respectfully care for our environment or we shall ultimately perish. The choise is ours.

In this book we have seen that medicine has some deeply seated roots in early ethical traditions. Some of these ethical notions, like that of man's harmony-disharmony with nature and natural law have often been obscured or denied but in view of the impending ecological and ideological crises, they take on important new values and meanings. We have seen how the Hippocratic traditions have expanded somewhat, especially in the past century, as the need for social awareness has increased and the physician has moved away somewhat from the old and traditional paternalistic role toward one of empathetic support; however, this is still far from optimal.

I indicated that these ancient ethical traditions gradually fused with the idea of the professional person and I suggested a device or model that would graphically represent the elements of the Hippocratic Legacy. The base or hub is *philia* or brotherly love from which radiate competence, responsibility, discipline, and service. Responsibility must always balance the autonomy that is a characteristic of the professional person. I took considerable space to explain that organized medicine was subject to the same ethical constraints as individual physicians but from an examination of the record it was clear that these ethical requirements have not always been met. It appears now that organized medicine in this country will become a more confessed political structure that will be the last bastion of those who champion private practice as the preferred model of medical care. This, of course, will take it far from its original purposes of improving educational standards and establishing ethical conduct. Throughout this book I have attempted to show that medicine's Hippocratic Legacy demands a much more comprehensive model of health care from physicians than the private practice, fee-for-service one: in the former there would be pervasive concerns for service to society and a preventive approach to health care. It is regrettable that organized medicine did not furnish the initiative and leadership for this expanded role.

The medical profession has faltered in its tradition of discipline for insuring the competence and responsibility of each physician. Unless the tradition of responsibility can be more widely exercised, painful and clumsy legislation will be enacted. Physicians simply must be more accountable, preferably to their peers, in the context of *philia* and those who are impaired must be exposed and helped in the same context; it can be done and is being done in some locales.

The medical profession must help find better solutions to the social problems which help produce disease; these problems include ruinous life styles, disruption of family-centered life, and attitudes toward the elderly and chronically ill. A much more active role in controlling the costs of medical care must be played or the present "system" will collapse. Pervasive changes are in order for American medicine which, in some cases, may not be optimal or desirable unless more suitable reforms are initiated by the profession.

The ethical physician is the one whose practice is based on *philia* and this physician will protect the rights of the patient and live an exemplary life to which the community may look as a model.

An important approach to obtaining quality physicians is a better selection of students with an improved educational ambience which requires a better faculty. A humane, competent, and ethical faculty which offers empathetic support to humane and ethical students can produce superior physicians who are wholly competent. Physicians must be realistically trained in the principles of health maintenance and prepared to teach the public in principles of self-care and healthful life styles.

Physicians may best fulfill the Hippocratic Legacy within the context of stewardship. The medical steward deals with ethical problems in medicine by the situation approach, using the Hippocratic Legacy for guidelines, but asking only within the context of *philia* love what is best for the person or persons involved. Although such an approach is concerned with consequences rather than inflexible rules, there is evidence that the situation approach is entirely in harmony with natural law and an important part of genetic programming. Love is basic to human life and therefore is one of the Creator's gifts and must be a part of the natural order.

Without *philia* we cannot develop the wisdom we need to successfully manage the expanding technology at our disposal and continue to improve the quality of life. The ultimate choice is destruction or remaining in harmonious balance with our biosphere.

APPENDIX A _____

AMERICAN HOSPITAL ASSOCIATION: A PATIENT'S BILL OF RIGHTS

1. The patient has the right to considerate and respectful care.
2. The patient has the right to obtain from his physician complete current information concerning his diagnosis, treatment, and prognosis in terms the patient can be reasonably expected to understand. When it is not medically advisable to give such information to the patient, the information should be made available to an appropriate person in his behalf. He has the right to know, by name, the physician responsible for coordinating his care.
3. The patient has the right to receive from his physician information necessary to give informed consent prior to the start of any procedure and/or treatment. Except in emergencies, such information for informed consent should include but not necessarily be limited to the specific procedure and/or treatment, the medically significant risks involved, and the probable duration of incapacitation. Where medically significant alternatives for care or treatment exist, or when the patient requests information concerning medical alternatives, the patient has the right to such information. The patient also has the right to know the name of the person responsible for the procedures and/or treatment.

4. The patient has the right to refuse treatment to the extent permitted by law and to be informed of the medical consequences of his action.

5. The patient has the right to every consideration of his privacy concerning his own medical care program. Case discussion, consultation, examination, and treatment are confidential and should be conducted discreetly. Those not directly involved in his care must have the permission of the patient to be present.

6. The patient has the right to expect that all communications and records pertaining to his care should be treated as confidential.

7. The patient has the right to expect that within its capacity a hospital must make reasonable response to the request of a patient for services. The hospital must provide evaluation, service, and/or referral as indicated by the urgency of the case. When medically permissable, a patient may be transferred to another facility only after he has received complete information and explanation concerning the needs for and alternatives to such a transfer. The institution to which the patient is to be transferred must first have accepted the patient for transfer.

8. The patient has the right to obtain information as to any relationship of his hospital to other health care and educational institutions insofar as his care is concerned. The patient has the right to obtain information as to the existence of any professional relationships among individuals, by name, who are treating him.

9. The patient has the right to be advised if the hospital proposes to engage in or perform human experimentation affecting his care or treatment. The patient has the right to refuse to participate in research projects.

10. The patient has the right to expect reasonable continuity of care. He has the right to know in advance what appointment times and physicians are available and where. The patient has the right to expect that the hospital will provide a mechanism whereby he is informed by his physician or a delegate of the physician of the patient's continuing health care requirements following discharge.

11. The patient has the right to examine and receive an explanation of his bill regardless of source of payment.

12. The patient has the right to know what hospital rules and regulations apply to his conduct as a patient.

No catalog of rights can guarantee for the patient the kind of treatment he has a right to expect. A hospital has many functions to perform, including the prevention and treatment of disease, the education of both health professionals and patients, and the conduct of clinical research. All these activities must be conducted with an overriding concern for the patient, and, above all, the recognition of his dignity as a human being. Success in achieving this recognition assures success in the defense of the rights of the patient.

AMERICAN MEDICAL ASSOCIATION: PRINCIPLES OF MEDICAL ETHICS VERSION OF 1957

PREAMBLE

These principles are intended to aid physicians individually and collectively in maintaining a high level of ethical conduct. They are not laws but standards by which a physician may determine the propriety of his conduct in his relationship with patients, with colleagues, with members of allied professions, and with the public.

SECTION I

The principal objective of the medical profession is to render service to humanity with full respect for the dignity of man. Physicians should merit the confidence of patients entrusted to their care, rendering to each a full measure of service and devotion.

SECTION II

Physicians should strive continually to improve medical knowledge and skill, and should make available to their patients and colleagues the benefits of their professional attainments.

SECTION III

A physician should practice a method of healing founded on a scientific basis; and he should not voluntarily associate professionally with anyone who violates this principle.

SECTION IV

The medical profession should safeguard the public and itself against physicians deficient in moral character or professional competence. Physicians should observe all laws, uphold the dignity and honor of the profession and accept its self-imposed disciplines. They should expose, without hesitation, illegal or unethical conduct of fellow members of the profession.

SECTION V

A physician may choose whom he will serve. In an emergency, however, he should render service to the best of his ability. Having undertaken the care of a patient, he may not neglect him; and unless he has been discharged he may discontinue his services only after giving adequate notice. He should not solicit patients.

SECTION VI

A physician should not dispose of his services under terms or conditions which tend to interfere with or impair the free and complete exercise of his medical judgment and skill or tend to cause a deterioration of the quality of medical care.

SECTION VII

In the practice of medicine a physician should limit the source of his professional income to medical services actually rendered by him, or under his supervision, to his patients. His fee should be commensurate with the services rendered and the patient's ability to pay. He should neither pay nor receive a commission for referral of patients. Drugs, remedies or appliances may be dispensed or supplied by the physician provided it is in the best interests of the patient.

SECTION VIII

A physician should seek consultation upon request; in doubtful or difficult cases; or whenever it appears that the quality of medical service may be enhanced thereby.

SECTION IX

A physician may not reveal the confidences entrusted to him in the course of medical attendance, or the deficiencies he may observe in the character of patients, unless he is required to do so by law or unless it becomes necessary in order to protect the welfare of the individual or of the community.

SECTION X

The honored ideals of the medical profession imply that the responsibilities of the physician extend not only to the individual, but also to society where these responsibilities deserve his interest and participation in activities which have the purpose of improving both the health and the well-being of the individual and the community.

AMERICAN MEDICAL ASSOCIATION: PRINCIPLES OF MEDICAL ETHICS REVISION OF 1980

PREAMBLE

The medical profession has long subscribed to a body of ethical statements developed primarily for the benefit of the patient. As a member of this profession, a physician must recognize responsibility not only to patients, but also to society, to other health professionals, and to self. The following Principles adopted by the American Medical Association are not laws, but standards of conduct which define the essentials of honorable behavior for the physician.

I. A physician shall be dedicated to providing competent medical service with compassion and respect for human dignity.

II. A physician shall deal honestly with patients and colleagues, and strive to expose those physicians deficient in character or competence, or who engage in fraud or deception.

III. A physician shall respect the law and also recognize a responsibility to seek changes in those requirements which are contrary to the best interests of the patient.

IV. A physician shall respect the rights of patients, of colleagues, and of other health professionals, and shall safeguard patient confidences with the constraints of the law.

V. A physician shall continue to study, apply, and advance scientific knowledge, make relevant information available to patients, colleagues, and the public, obtain consultation, and use the talents of other health professionals when indicated.

VI. A physician shall, in the provision of appropriate patient care, except in emergencies, be free to choose whom to serve, with whom to associate, and the environment in which to provide medical services.

VII. A physician shall recognize a responsibility to participate in activities contributing to an improved community.

CALIFORNIA NATURAL DEATH ACT CHAPTER 3.9

7185. This act shall be known and may be cited as the Natural Death Act.

7186. The Legislature finds that adult persons have the fundamental right to control the decisions relating to the rendering of their own medical care, including the decision to have life-sustaining procedures withheld or withdrawn in instances of a terminal condition.

The Legislature further finds that modern medical technology has made possible the artificial prolongation of human life beyond natural limits.

The Legislature further finds that, in the interest of protecting individual autonomy, such prolongation of life for persons with a terminal condition may cause loss of patient dignity and unnecessary pain and suffering, while providing nothing medically necessary or beneficial to the patient.

The Legislature further finds that there exists considerable uncertainty in the medical and legal professions as to the legality of terminating the use or application of life-sustaining procedures where the patient has voluntarily and in sound mind evidenced a desire that such procedures be withheld or withdrawn.

In recognition of the dignity and privacy which patients have a right to expect, the Legislature hereby declares that the laws of the State of California shall recognize the right of an adult person to make a written directive instructing his physician to withhold or withdraw life-sustaining procedures in the event of a terminal condition.

7187. The following definitions shall govern the construction of this chapter:

(a) "Attending physician" means the physician selected by, or assigned to, the patient who has primary responsibility for the treatment and care of the patient.

(b) "Directive" means a written document voluntarily executed by the declarant in accordance with the requirements of Section 7188. The directive, or a copy of the directive, shall be made part of the patient's medical records.

(c) "Life-sustaining procedure" means any medical procedure or intervention which utilizes mechanical or other artificial means to sustain, restore, or supplant a vital function, which, when applied to a qualified patient, would serve only to artifically prolong the moment of death and where, in the judgment of the attending physician, death is imminent whether or not such procedures are utilized.

(c) "Life-sustaining procedure" shall not include the administration of medication or the performance of any medical procedure deemed necessary to alleviate pain.

(d) "Physician" means a physician and surgeon licensed by the Board of Medical Quality Assurance or the Board of Osteopathic Examiners.

(e) "Qualified patient" means a patient diagnosed and certified in writing to be afflicted with a terminal condition by two physicians, one of whom shall be the attending physician, who have personally examined the patient.

(f) "Terminal condition" means an incurable condition caused by injury, disease, or illness, which, regardless of the application of life-sustaining procedures, would, within reasonable medical judgment, produce death, and where the application of life-sustaining procedures serve only to postpone the moment of death of the patient.

7188. Any adult person may execute a directive directing the withholding or withdrawal of life-sustaining procedures in a terminal condition. The directive shall be signed by the declarant in the presence of two witnesses not related to the declarant by blood or marriage and who would not be entitled to any portion of the estate of the declarant upon his decease under any will of the declarant or codicil thereto then existing or, at the time of the directive, by operation of law then existing. In addition, a witness to a directive shall not be the attending physician, an employee of the attending physician or a health facility in which the declarant is a patient, or any person who has a claim against any portion of the estate of the declarant upon his decease at the time of the execution of the directive. The directive shall be in the following form:

DIRECTIVE TO PHYSICIANS

Directive made this _____ day of _____ (month, year).

I _____, being of sound mind, willfully, and voluntarily make known my desire that my life shall not be artificially prolonged under the circumstances set forth below, do hereby declare:

1. If at any time I should have an incurable injury, disease, or illness certified to be a terminal condition by two physicians, and where the application of life-sustaining procedures would serve only to artificially prolong the moment of my death and where my physician determines that my death is imminent whether or not life-sustaining procedures are utilized, I direct that such procedures be withheld or withdrawn, and that I be permitted to die naturally.

2. In the absence of my ability to give directions regarding the use of such life-sustaining procedures, it is my intention that this directive shall be honored by my family and physician(s) as the final expression of my legal right to refuse medical or surgical treatment and accept the consequences from such refusal.

3. If I have been diagnosed as pregnant and that diagnosis is known to my physician, this directive shall have no force or effect during the course of my pregnancy.

4. I have been diagnosed and notified at least 14 days ago as having a terminal condition by _____, M.D., whose address is _____, and whose telephone number is _____. I understand that if I have not filled in the physician's name and address, it shall be presumed that I did not have a terminal condition when I made out this directive.

5. This directive shall have no force or effect five years from the date filled in above.

6. I understand the full import of this directive and I am emotionally and mentally competent to make this directive.

Signed _____

City, County and State of Residence _____

The declarant has been personally known to me and I believe him or her to be of sound mind.

Witness _____

Witness _____

7188.5. A directive shall have no force or effect if the declarant is a patient in a skilled nursing facility as defined in subdivision (c) of Section 1250 at the time the directive is executed unless one of the two witnesses to the directive is a patient advocate or ombudsman as may be designated by the State Department of Aging for this purpose pursuant to any other applicable provision of law. The patient advocate or ombudsman shall have the same qualifications as a witness under Section 7188.

The intent of this section is to recognize that some patients in skilled nursing facilities may be so insulated from a voluntary decision-making role, by virtue of the custodial nature of their care, as to require special assurance that they are capable of willfully and voluntarily executing a directive.

7189. (a) A directive may be revoked at any time by the declarant, without regard to his mental state or competency, by any of the following methods:

(1) By being canceled, defaced, obliterated, or burnt, torn, or otherwise destroyed by the declarant or by some person in his presence and by his direction.

(2) By a written revocation of the declarant expressing his intent to revoke, signed and dated by the declarant. Such revocation shall become effective only upon communication to the attending physician by the declarant or by a person acting on behalf of the declarant. The attending physician shall record in the patient's medical record the time and date when he received notification of the written revocation.

(3) By a verbal expression by the declarant of his intent to revoke the directive. Such revocation shall become effective only upon communication to the attending physician by the declarant or by a person acting on behalf of the declarant. The attending physician shall record in the patient's medical record the time, date, and place of the revocation and the time, date, and place, if different, of when he received notification of the revocation.

(b) There shall be no criminal or civil liability on the part of any person for failure to act upon a revocation made pursuant to this section unless that person has actual knowledge of the revocation.

7189.5. A directive shall be effective for five years from the date of execution thereof unless sooner revoked in a manner prescribed in Section 7189. Nothing in this chapter shall be construed to prevent a declarant from reexecuting a directive at any time in accordance with the formalities of Section 7188, including reexecution subsequent to a diagnosis of a terminal condition. If the declarant has executed more than one directive, such time shall be determined from the date of execution of the last directive known to the attending physician. If the declarant becomes comatose or is rendered incapable of communicating with the attending physician, the directive shall remain in effect for the duration of the comatose condition or until such time as the declarant's condition renders him or her able to communicate with the attending physician.

7190. No physician or health facility which, acting in accordance with the requirements of this chapter, causes the withholding or withdrawal of life-sustaining procedures from a qualified patient, shall be subject to civil liability therefrom. No licensed health professional, acting under the direction of a physician, who participates in the withholding or withdrawal of life sustaining procedures in accordance with the provisions of this chapter shall be subject to any civil liability. No physician, or licensed health professional acting under the direction of a physician, who participates in the withholding or withdrawal of life-sustaining procedures in accordance with the provisions of this chapter shall be guilty of any criminal act or of unprofessional conduct.

7191. (a) Prior to effecting a withholding or withdrawal of life-sustaining procedures from a qualified patient pursuant to the directive, the attending physician shall determine that the directive complies with Section 7188, and, if the patient is mentally competent, that the directive and all steps proposed by the attending physician to be undertaken are in accord with the desires of the qualified patient.

(b) If the declarant was a qualified patient at least 14 days prior to executing or reexecuting the directive, the directive shall be conclusively presumed, unless revoked, to be the directions of the patient regarding the withholding or withdrawal of life-sustaining procedures. No physician, and no licensed health professional acting under the direction of a physician, shall be criminally or civilly liable for failing to effectuate the directive of the qualified patient pursuant to this subdivision. A failure by a physician to effectuate the directive of a qualified patient pursuant to this division shall constitute unprofessional conduct if the physician refuses to make the necessary arrangements, or fails to take the necessary steps, to effect the transfer of the qualified patient to another physician who will effectuate the directive of the qualified patient.

(c) If the declarant becomes a qualified patient subsequent to executing the directive, and has not subsequently reexecuted the directive, the attending physician may give weight to the directive as evidence of the patient's directions regarding the withholding or withdrawal of life-sustaining procedures and may consider other factors, such as information from the affected family or the nature of the patient's illness, injury, or disease, in determining whether the totality of circumstances known to the attending physician justify effectuating the directive. No physician, and no licensed health professional acting under the direction of a physician, shall be criminally or civilly liable for failing to effectuate the directive of the qualified patient pursuant to this subdivision.

7192. (a) The withholding or withdrawal of life-sustaining procedures from a qualified patient in accordance with the provisions of this chapter shall not, for any purpose, constitute a suicide.

(b) The making of a directive pursuant to Section 7188 shall not restrict, inhibit, or impair in any manner the sale, procurement, or issuance of any policy of life insurance, nor shall it be deemed to modify the terms of an existing policy of life insurance. No policy of life insurance shall be legally impaired or invalidated in any manner by the withholding or withdrawal of life-sustaining procedures from an insured qualified patient, notwithstanding any term of the policy to the contrary.

(c) No physician, health facility, or other health provider, and no health care service plan, insurer issuing disability insurance, self-insured employee welfare benefit plan or nonprofit hospital service plan, shall require any person to execute a directive as a condition for being insured for, or receiving, health care services.

7193. Nothing in this chapter shall impair or supersede any legal right or legal responsibility which any person may have to effect the withholding or withdrawal of life-sustaining procedures in any lawful manner. In such respect the provisions of this chapter are cumulative.

7194. Any person who willfully conceals, cancels, defaces, obliterates, or damages the directive of another without such declarant's consent shall be guilty of a misdemeanor. Any person who, except where justified or excused by law, falsifies or forges the directive of another, or willfully conceals or withholds personal knowledge of a revocation as provided in Section 7189, with the intent to cause a withholding or withdrawal of life sustaining procedures contrary to the wishes of the declarant, and thereby, because of any such act, directly causes life-sustaining procedures to be withheld or withdrawn and death to thereby be hastened, shall be subject to prosecution for unlawful homicide as provided in Chapter 1 (commending with Section 197) of Title 8 of Part 1 of the Penal Code.

7195. Nothing in this chapter shall be construed to condone, authorize, or approve mercy killing, or to permit any affirmative or deliberate act or ommission to end life other than to permit the natural process of dying as provided in this chapter.

SEC. 2. If any provision of this act or the application thereof to any person or circumstances is held invalid, such invalidity shall not affect other provisions or applications of the act which can be given effect without the invalid provision or application, and to this end the provisions of the act are severable.

SEC. 3. Notwithstanding Section 2231 of the Revenue and Taxation Code, there shall be no reimbursement pursuant to this section nor shall there be any appropriation made by this act because the Legislature recognizes that during any legislative session a variety of changes to laws relating to crimes and infractions may cause both increased and decreased costs to local government entities and school districts which, in the aggregate, do not result in significant identifiable cost changes.

CONCERN FOR DYING: A LIVING WILL

TO MY FAMILY, MY PHYSICIAN, MY LAWYER, AND ALL OTHERS WHOM IT MAY CONCERN

Death is as much a reality as birth, growth, maturity and old age—it is the one certainty of life. If the time comes when I can no longer take part in decisions for my own future, let this statement stand as an expression of my wishes and directions, while I am still of sound mind.

If at such a time the situation should arise in which there is no reasonable expectation of my recovery from extreme physical or mental disability, I direct that I be allowed to die and not be kept alive by medications, artificial means or "heroic measures." I do, however, ask that medication be mercifully administered to me to alleviate suffering even though this may shorten my remaining life.

This statement is made after careful consideration and is in accordance with my strong convictions and beliefs. I want the wishes and directions here expressed carried out to the extent permitted by law. Insofar as they are not legally enforceable, I hope that those to whom this Will is addressed will regard themselves as morally bound by these provisions.

Signed _____

Date _____

Witness _____

Witness _____

Copies of this request have been given to _____

_____

_____

_____

Reprinted with Permission from

Concern for Dying
250 West 57 Street
New York, N.Y. 10107

WORLD MEDICAL ASSOCIATION: DECLARATION OF GENEVA

A PLEDGE SUGGESTED AS A DEDICATION OF THE PHYSICIAN TO HIS PROFESSION OF SERVICE ADOPTED BY THE GENERAL ASSEMBLY OF THE WORLD MEDICAL ASSOCIATION IN GENEVA, SEPTEMBER, 1948

At the time of being admitted as Member of the Medical Profession.

I solemnly pledge myself to consecrate my life to the service of humanity.

I will give to my teachers the respect and gratitude which is their due;

I will practice my profession with conscience and dignity;

The health of my patient will be my first consideration;

I will respect the secrets which are confided in me;

I will maintain by all the means in my power, the honor and the noble traditions of the medical profession;

My colleagues will be my brothers;

I will not permit considerations of religion, nationality, race, party politics or social standing to intervene between my duty and my patient;

I will maintain the utmost respect for human life, from the time of conception; even under threat, I will not use my medical knowledge contrary to the laws of humanity.

I make these promises solemnly, freely and upon my honor.

WORLD MEDICAL ASSOCIATION: DECLARATION OF HELSINKI

RECOMMENDATIONS GUIDING DOCTORS IN CLINICAL RESEARCH

Introduction

It is the mission of the doctor to safeguard the health of the people. His knowledge and conscience are dedicated to the fulfillment of this mission.

The Declaration of Geneva of the World Medical Association binds the doctor with the words: "The health of my patient will be my first consideration" and the International Code of Medical Ethics which declares that "Any act or advice which could weaken physical or mental resistance of a human being may be used only in his interest."

Because it is essential that the results of laboratory experiments be applied to human beings to further scientific knowledge and to help suffering humanity, the World Medical Association has prepared the following recommendations as a guide to each doctor in clinical research. It must be stressed that the standards as drafted are only a guide to physicians all over the world. Doctors are not relieved from criminal, civil and ethical responsibilities under the laws of their own countries.

In the field of clinical research a fundamental distinction must be recognized between clinical research in which the aim is essentially therapeutic for a patient, and the clinical research, the essential object of which is purely scientific and without therapeutic value to the person subjected to the research.

I) Basic Principles

1) Clinical research must conform to the moral and scientific principles that justify medical research and should be based on laboratory and animal experiments or other scientifically established facts.

2) Clinical research should be conducted only by scientifically qualified persons and under the supervision of a qualified medical man.

3) Clinical research cannot legitimately be carried out unless the importance of the objective is in proportion to the inherent risk to the subject.

4) Every clinical research project should be preceded by careful assessment of inherent risks in comparison to forseeable benefits to the subject or to others.

5) Special caution should be exercised by the doctor in performing clinical research in which the personality of the subject is liable to be altered by drugs or experimental procedure.

II) Clinical Research Combined with Professional Care

1) In the treatment of the sick person, the doctor must be free to use a new therapeutic measure, if in his judgment it offers hope of saving life, reestablishing health, or alleviating suffering.

If at all possible, consistent with patient psychology, the doctor should obtain the patient's freely given consent after the patient has been given a full explanation. In case of legal incapacity, consent should also be procured from the legal guardian; in case of physical incapacity the permission of the legal guardian replaces that of the patient.

2) The doctor can combine clinical research with professional care, the objective being the acquisition of new medical knowledge, only to the extent that clinical research is justified by its therapeutic value for the patient.

III) Non-Therapeutic Clinical Research

1) In the purely scientific application of clinical research carried out on a human being, it is the duty of the doctor to remain the protector of the life and health of that person on whom clinical research is being carried out.

2) The nature, the purpose and the risk of clinical research must be explained to the subject by the doctor.

3a) Clinical research on a human being cannot be undertaken without his free consent after he has been informed; if he is legally incompetent, the consent of the legal guardian should be procured.

3b) The subject of clinical research should be in such a mental, physical and legal state as to be able to exercise fully his power of choice.

3c) Consent should, as a rule, be obtained in writing. However, the responsibility for clinical research always remains with the research worker; it never falls on the subject even after consent is obtained.

4a) The investigator must respect the right of each individual to safeguard his personal integrity, especially if the subject is in a dependent relationship to the investigator.

4b) At any time during the course of clinical research the subject or his guardian should be free to withdraw permission for research to be continued.

The investigator or the investigating team should discontinue the research if in his or their judgment, it may, if continued, be harmful to the individual.

VAN RENSSELAER POTTER: A BIOETHICAL CREED FOR INDIVIDUALS

1. *Belief*: I accept the need for remedial action in a world beset with crisis.

Commitment: I will work with others to improve the formulation of my beliefs, to evolve additional credos, and to unite in a worldwide movement that will make possible the survival and improved development of the human species in harmony with the natural environment.

2. *Belief*: I accept the fact that the future survival and development of mankind, both culturally and biologically, is strongly conditioned by man's present activities and plans.

Commitment: I will try to live my own life and to influence the lives of others so as to promote the evolution of a better world for future generations of mankind, and I will try to avoid actions that would jeopardize their future.

3. *Belief*: I accept the uniqueness of each individual and his instinctive need to contribute to the betterment of some larger unit of society in a way that is compatible with the long-range needs of society.

Commitment: I will try to listen to the reasoned viewpoint of others whether from a minority or a majority, and I will recognize the role of emotional commitment in producing effective action.

4. *Belief*: I accept the inevitability of some human suffering that must result from the natural disorder in biological creatures and in the physical world, but I do not passively accept the suffering that results from man's inhumanity to man.

Commitment: I will try to face my own problems with dignity and courage, I will try to assist my fellow men when they are afflicted, and I will work toward the goal of eliminating needless suffering among mankind as a whole.

5. *Belief*: I accept the finality of death as a necessary part of life, I affirm the veneration for life, my belief in the botherhood of man, and my belief that I have an obligation to future generations of man.

Commitment: I will try to live in a way that will benefit the lives of my fellow men now and in time to come and be remembered favorably by those who survive me.

Van Rensselaer Potter, BIOETHICS: Bridge to the Future, copyright 1971. Reprinted by permission of Prentice-Hall, Inc., Englewood Cliffs, New Jersey.

NOTES

CHAPTER 1

1. P. L. Entralgo, *Doctor and Patient* (New York: McGraw-Hill, 1969), p. 53.

2. N. B. Etziony, *The Physician's Creed* (Springfield: Charles Thomas, 1973), pp. 15-20.

3. Ralph Major, *A History of Medicine* (Springfield: Charles Thomas, 1954), pp. 20-101.

4. *Old Testament Apocrypha*, Ecclesiasticus 38:1-4, New English Bible.

5. P. L. Entralgo, *Mind and Body* (London: Harvill, 1955), Chapter III; L. Edelstein, "The Professional Ethics of the Greek Physician," *Bulletin of the History of Medicine* 30 (1956):391-419.

6. L. Edelstein, "The Hippocratic Oath," *Bulletin of the History of Medicine* 1 (1943) supplement.

7. This information comes from Chinese writings of the eighth century A.D., but probably originated earlier. This ethical heritage is certainly being carried on by mainland China today. See the book review on *Medical Ethics in Imperial China* by Robert K. Veatch, *Journal of the A.M.A.* 242 (September 28, 1979):1411.

8. Edelstein, "The Hippocratic Oath," p. 64.

9. Major, *A History of Medicine*, pp. 118-21.

10. Major, *A History of Medicine*, p. 121.

11. The two great commandments came from that part of the Old Testament known as the Law or Pentateuch and are found in Deuteronomy 6:5 and Leviticus 1 19:18. Jesus quotes these in Matthew 22:37 f. and states that one is like the other. See also Galatians 5:14, Romans 13:9, and James 2:8. Jesus also stated that he had no intention of destroying the Law but to give it new life in Matthew 5:17.

12. Entralgo, *Mind and Body*, p. 68

13. Joseph Fletcher, *Situation Ethics* (Philadelphia: Westminster, 1966) p. 27-28.

14. A. Bar-Sela and H. E. Hoff, "Isaac Israel's Fifty Admonitions to the Physicians," *J. of the History of Medicine and Allied Sciences* 17 (1962). This article, with several others, is reprinted in the book, *Legacies in Ethics and Medicine*, edited by Chester Burns. This annotated collection is very helpful for tracing the development of medical ethics in the West.

15. M. Levey, "Medical Deontology in 9th Century Islam," *J. History of Medicine and Allied Sciences*, 21 (Oct. 1966):385.

16. Ibid.

17. D. W. Amundsen, "The Liability of the Greek Physician in Classical Greek Legal Theory and Practice", *J. History of Medicine and Allied Sciences* vol. 32, no. 2 (April 1977):172-203.

18. For an excellent documentary history of the legal regulation of medical practice, please refer to Chester Burns, ed., *Legacies in Law and Medicine*, (New York: Science History Publications, 1977).

CHAPTER 2

1. There is some evidence that nursing is the oldest profession. It is comforting to think that caring may have come before commerce.

2. L. Edelstein, "The Professional Ethics of the Greek Physician," *Bulletin of the History of Medicine,* 30 (1956): 408ff.

3. Wilbert E. Moore, *The Professions: Roles and Rules* (New York: Russell Sage Foundation, 1970). pp. 7-17.

4. *Opinions and Report of the Judicial Council of the AMA* (Chicago: American Medical Association, 1971), p. vi.

5. See "Text of A.M.A.'s New Principles of Ethics," *American Medical News* (August 18, 1980), p. 9.

6. Charles Dickens's *Hard Times* vividly portrays the temper and conditions of the life of the poor in early nineteenth century England.

7. It comes as a surprise to some that we have social medicine programs now. We have had Medicaid and Medicare programs since 1965, we have the free medical care provided our Armed Forces, the Veterans Administration, and various state institutions caring for the mentally incompetent.

8. Chester Burns, ed., *Legacies in Ethics and Medicine,* (New York: Science History Publications, 1977), p. 293.

CHAPTER 4

1. *Medical Education in the United States and Canada,* Carnegie Foundation for the Advancement of Teaching, Bulletin no. 4 (New York, 1910).

2. "The A. M. A., Power, Purpose, and Politics in Organized Medicine," *Yale Law Journal* 63 (May 1954):970.

3. James G. Burrow, *A. M. A.: Voice of American Medicine* (Baltimore: Johns Hopkins Press, 1963), pp. 286, 322.

4. Grace Ziem, "Medical Education Since Flexner," *Health/PAC Bulletin* 76 (May/June 1977):8-14.

5. James G. Burrow, *Organized Medicine in the Progressive Era: The Move Toward Monopoly,* (Baltimore: Johns Hopkins Press, 1977). pp. 140-43.

6. Ruth Mulvay Harmer, *American Medical Avarice* (New York: Abelard-Schuman, 1975), p. 20.

7. From Resolutions, AMA, June 1973, p. 337.

8. Socialized medicine is a reality in the form of current Medicaid and Medicare programs with an estimated cost in 1980 of twenty billion dollars. In addition, there is free medical care to the armed forces personnel and their dependents.

9. Saul Krugman and Samuel Katz, "Childhood Immunization Procedures," *Journal of the A.M.A.* 237 (May 16, 1977):2228-30.

10. *The Medical Letter*, 18, no. 25 (December 3, 1976):108.

11. *Report of the Secretary's Commission on Medical Malpractice*, DHEW Publication No. (OS) 73-89 1973, Appendix, p. 50.

12. "The Influence of the Manpower Study of SOSUSS on Graduate Education in Surgery," *Bulletin of the American College of Surgeons* (February/March 1976).

13. Eugene McCarthy and Geraldine Widmer, "Effects of Screening by Consultants on Recommended Elective Surgical Procedures," *New England Journal of Medicine* 291 (December 19, 1974):1331-35. This report touched off a controversy which has been boiling ever since. A more recent report stated that on a simple "yes or no" basis, the second consultant said "no" in 24 percent of the cases but that "detailed analysis" showed a firm rejection in only 8 percent of the cases. (W. Paris, E. Salsberg, and L. Berenson, "An Analysis of Non-confirmation Rates," *Journal of the American Medical Association* 242 (November 30, 1979):2424-27. Even more arresting is an article in the *American Medical News* for November 9, 1979 (also published by the AMA) which states that a new study done by the AMA's Surgical Criteria Project for the United States Department of HEW will show that only 1 percent of the surgical cases in its series could be termed unnecessary. Why the HEW chose the AMA to conduct this study is unclear. Meanwhile, HEW continues to push for second opinions in all cases of elective surgery in its Medicaid and Medicare programs.

14. *American Medical News*, December 13, 1976.

15. *American Medical News*, January 31, 1977.

16. "The American Medical Association and the American Doctor: Sharing a Common Goal," AMA pamphlet, n.d., ca. 1973.

17. "The A.M.A., Power, Purpose, and Politics in Organized Medicine," p. 1018.

18. *American Medical News*, March 14, 1980, p. 7. This article reports that in a 1979 Gallup poll only 30 percent of people queried thought that AMA policies and actions were clearly in the public interest; a 9 percent decrease since a similar 1976 poll.

CHAPTER 5

1. H. R. Kaplan, "The Fee-for-Service System," in *Humanistic Perspectives in Medical Ethics*, ed. M. B. Visscher (Buffalo: Prometheus Books, 1972), pp. 135-62. There have been a good number of articles in recent years which have pointed out that the temptation to abuse cannot be removed from such a system.

2. *Santa Fe New Mexican*, April 26, 1976.

3. Robert Stevens and Rosemary Stevens, *Welfare Medicine in America* (New York: The Free Press, 1974), 194ff.

4. George Crile, Jr., "The Surgeon's Dilemma," *Harper's*, May 1975, pp. 30-38.

5. Bhopinder S. Bolaria, "Professionalism Among American and English Physicians" (Ph.D. diss., Washington State University, 1967)

6. Various contributors, "California's Medi-Cal Copayment Experiment," *Medical Care* vol. 12 no. 12 supplement (Dec. 1974): 1051-58.

CHAPTER 6

1. Until just recently it was possible to practice in a few states without any postgraduate training (internship or residency years).

2. According to a survey made by *Medical World News* of disciplinary actions taken by state boards for the period 1969-73 California led the list with 245 revocations out of some 33,606 physicians in patient care. New York had only 14 revocations out of some 36,161 physicians in patient care and in 16 states there were no revocations. Missouri, South Carolina, Pennsylvania, and Louisiana did not furnish any information. See *Medical World News*, March 15, 1974, p. 68. Since 1974 there has been a growing trend for more disciplinary actions.

3. "Impaired Physicians: Medicine Bites the Bullet," *Medical World News*, July 24, 1978. pp. 40-51; "Impaired M.D. Reporting Guide Issued," *American Medical News*, February 8, 1980. The latter article discusses the new guidelines of the California Medical Association.

4. A current medical audit program to study outcome is known as the Performance Evaluation Procedure and has been instituted by the Joint Commission for the Accreditation of Hospitals as a requirement for accreditation. There have been problems in this approach. See E. William Rosenberg; "Medical Audit JCAH-Style," *JAMA*, 237 no. 18 (May 2, 1977):1935-7.

5. *New York Times*, January 30, 1976, p. 1f.

6. American Medical Association, *Medical Ethics and Discipline Manual*, 1966, p 4.

7. Derbyshire, Robert C. "Medical Ethics and Discipline," *Journal of the A.M.A.* 228 (April 1, 1974):61.

8. *Report of the Medical Disciplinary Committee to the Board of Trustees of the American Medical Association*, June, 1961.

9. *Medical World News*, March 15, 1974, p. 62-72.

10. *American Medical News*, July 11, 1977, p. 22.

11. *American Medical News*, Sept. 8, 1975, p. 1.

12. Crosby, William H. "Lead-contaminated Health Food", *Journal of the A.M.A.* vol. 237 no. 24 (June 13, 1978):2627-29.

CHAPTER 7

1. Thomas Szasz, *The Theology of Medicine* (Baton Rouge: Louisiana State University Press, 1977). pp. xiii-xxii.

2. U.S. Congress, Senate, Special Committee on Aging, "Doctors in Nursing Homes: The Shunned Responsibility," Supporting Paper No. 3, *Nursing Care in the United States: Failure in Public Policy* (Washington, D.C.: Government Printing Office, 1975).

3. Matt. 25:40.

4. Matt. 25:14-30.

5. Joseph Fletcher, "Indicators of Humanhood: A Tentative Profile of Man," *The Hastings Center Report* vol. 2 no. 5 (November, 1972):1-4.

6. Joseph Fletcher, "Four Indicators of Humanhood," *The Hastings Center Report* vol. 4 no. 6 (December, 1974): 4-7.

7. Duvalier was actually a medical doctor who worked in Haitian public health for several years before entering politics.

8. Leroy Augenstein, *Come Let us Play God* (New York: Harper and Row, 1969). pp. 142-46.

9. *See* "Bimedical Ethics and the Shadow of Nazism" *Hastings Center Report* vol. 6 no. 4 (August, 1976): 8-10, supplement. report of a conference edited by Peter Steinfels and Carol Levine.

10. Franklin J. Evans, "The Right to Die—a Basic Constitutional Right," *Journal of Legal Medicine* vol. 5 no. 8 (August 1977):17-20.

11. The Uniform Anatomical Gift Act permits a person to leave certain parts or all of his body for use by the living (tissue for transplant, etc.) or for anatomical study.

12. Philip Slater, *The Pursuit of Loneliness* rev. ed. (Boston: Beacon Press, 1976), p. 21.

13. Marc Lappé, "Moral Obligations and the Fallacies of "Genetic Control," *Theological Studies* vol. 33 no. 3 (September 1972):411-427.

14. John Osmundsen, "We Are All Mutants—Preventive Genetic Medicine: A Growing Clinical Field Troubled by a Confusion of Ethicists," *Medical Dimensions* (February 1973), pp. 5-28.

15. For a good survey of the issues in genetic screening, abortion, and newborn euthanasia, see George H. Kieffer, *Bioethics: A Textbook of Issues* (Reading: Addison-Wesley, 1979).

16. "Let Defective Babies Die," *American Medical News,* January 10, 1977; "Would it Ever be Right to Directly Intervene to Kill a Self-sustaining Infant?" *Family Practice News* February 15, 1977, p. 1.

17. Jacqueline M. Nolan-Haley, "Defective Children, Their Parents, and the Death Decision," *Journal of Legal Medicine* (January 1976), pp. 9-14.

18. "Wrongful Life: A New Legal Concept," *Medical World News*, (December 13, 1976), p. 49.

19. Victor and Ruth Sidel, "Self-reliance and the Collective Good: Medicine in China," *Ethics and Health Policy*, Veatch and Branson, eds. (Cambridge, Mass.: Ballinger, 1976).

CHAPTER 8

1. W. Walter Menninger, "'Caring' as Part of Health Care Quality," *J.A.M.A.* vol. 234, no. 8 (November 27, 1975):836-37.

2. Donnie J. Self, "Patient Rights and Physician Responsibilities," *Social Issues in Health Care*, Donnie J. Self, ed. (Norfolk: Old Dominion University Foundation, 1977), pp. 85-91.

3. Robert M. Sade, "Medical Care as a Right: A Refutation," *New England Journal of Medicine* 285 (December 2, 1977):1288-92.

4. Daniel Callahan, "Health and Society: Some Ethical Imperatives," *Doing Better and Feeling Worse: Health in the United States*, John H. Knowles, ed. (New York: Norton, 1977), pp. 30-33.

5. Karl Bauman, Richard Udry, and Naomi Morris, "Changes in Women's Preferences for the Racial Composition of Medical Facilities, 1969-74," *A.J.P.H.* vol. 66, no. 3 (March 1976):284-86.

6. Marcel Fredericks, John Kosa, and Paul Mundy, "Willingness to Serve: the Medical Profession and Poverty Programs," *Social Science and Medicine* vol. 8, no. 1 (January 1974):51-57.

7. James Cantrell and Barry Eisenberg, "Policies to Influence the Spatial Distribution of Physicians," *Medical Care* vol. 14, no. 6 (June 1976):455-68.

8. C. H. William Ruhe, "The Private Sector Can Answer the Need," *Prism* 3 (February 1975):15.

9. Rosemary Stevens, "Muddle over Medical Manpower," *Prism* 3 (February 1975):10-12.

10. Robert Derbyshire, "Warm Bodies in White Coats," *Journal of the A.M.A.* 232 (June 9, 1975):1034-35.

11. Roger Politzer et al., "Foreign-Trained Physicians in American Medicine," *Medical Care* vol. 16 no. 8 (September 1978):611-27.

12. Robert Saywell et al., "A Performance Comparison: USMG-FMG Attending Physicians," *A.J.P.H.* vol. 69 no. 1 (January 1979):57-62; Robert Saywell et al., "A Performance Comparison: USMG-FMG House Staff Physicians," *A.J.P.H.* vol. 70 no. 1 (January 1980):23-28.

13. "HEW Foresees Plenty of M.D.'s in Next Decade," *American Medical News*, April 25, 1980.

14. In this connection it is interesting to examine the attitude of the AMA toward FMGs. The AMA has more or less tacitly approved the immigration of FMGs to this country as one way to solve the manpower problem and to divert public attention from the AMA's failure to correct the problem with American physicians. In December 1975 I wrote a letter for publication to the editor of the *A.M.A. News* stating my objections to the acceptance of 350 physicians from Viet Nam to this country and raising the question of whether they truly were political refugees. I also spoke to the problem of retraining these physicians for practice in this country at very high cost and marginal quality, adding that if we truly cared for the Vietnamese we would not have taken away 20 percent of their physicians. I received no answer, so two months later I wrote the executive secretary of the AMA and related the sequence of events to him adding that it had been charged that the AMA would seldom publish any views in opposition to its own, and I would like to report that this charge was not true by personal experience. More than two years later I have still not heard from Doctor Sammons, the executive secretary.

15. Howard Spiro, "Should the Medical Schools Care?" *New England Journal of Medicine* vol. 292 no. 15 (April 10, 1975):792-24.

16. Michael Counte and John Kimberly, "Issues in Family Practice," *Medical Care* vol. 16 no. 3 (March 1978):214-25.

17. Henry Wechsler, et al., "A Follow-up Study of Residents in Internal Medicine, Pediatrics, and Obstetrics-Gynecology Training Programs in Massachusetts," *New England Journal of Medicine* vol. 298 no. 1 (January 5, 1978): 15-21.

18. Curtis Seltzer, "Health Care by the Ton," *Health/PAC Bulletin* 79 (November-December 1977):p. 1ff.

19. Jonathan Metsch and James Veney, "Consumer Participation and Social Accountability," *Medical Care* vol. 14 no. 4 (April 1976):283-92.

20. Vicente Navarro, "The Political and Economic Determinants of Health Care in Rural America," *Inquiry* vol. 8 no. 2 (June 1976):111-121; Arnold Kaluzny and David Smith, "Inequality in Health Care Programs," *Medical Care* (October 12, 1974), pp. 860-70.

21. Daniel Zwick, "Some Accomplishments and Fundings of Neighborhood Health Centers," *Organizational Issues in the Delivery of Health Services*, Irving Zola, ed. (New York: Prodist, 1974), pp. 331-64.

22. Lu Ann Aday, "Economic and Noneconomic Barriers to the Use of Needed Medical Services," *Medical Care* vol. 13, no. 6 (June 1976):447-56.

23. Karen Davis, "Medicaid Payments and Utilization of Health Services by the Poor," *Inquiry* vol. 8, no. 2 (June 1976):122-35; *see also* "Ten Years of Medicare and Medicaid," *Medical World News*, (March 10, 1975), p. 60ff.

24. Frank E. Moss, "Through the Medicaid Mills," *Journal of Legal Medicine* vol. 5, no. 5 (May 1977):7-11.

25. ABC Television Special, "Medicine and Money," 1976.

26. Janet B. Mitchell and Jerry Cromwell, "Medicaid Mills: Fact or Fiction", *Health Care Financing Review*, Summer 1980. pp. 37-49.

27. Robert Stevens and Rosemary Stevens, *Welfare Medicine in America* (New York: Free Press, 1974), p. 198.

28. Mary Mendelson, *Tender Loving Greed* (New York: Vintage Books, 1975), Val Halamandaris and Frank Moss, *Too Old Too Sick Too Bad* (Germantown: Aspen, 1977). There are several publications dealing with the nursing home problem consisting of evidence gathered by the U.S. Senate Subcommittee on Long-Term Care. U. S. Congress, Senate, Special Committee on Aging, "Doctors in Nursing Homes: The Shunned Responsibility," Supporting Paper No. 3, *Nursing Care in the United States: Failure in Public Policy* (Washington, D.C.: Government Printing Office, 1975). There are nine supporting papers or separate booklets in this series. An earlier publication by the same committee consists of affidavits and letters from people with first-hand experience with some of the terrible conditions prevailing in these homes: *Trends in Long-Term Care*, Part 19B-Appendix.

29. Robert Brook et al., "Controlling the Use and Cost of Medical Services," *Medical Care* vol. 16 no. 9 supplement (September 1978):75.

30. "Forty Million Poor Lack Health Coverage," *American Medical News*, January 7, 1977.

31. "Practicing M.D.'s Being Taught about Costs," *American Medical News*, April 25, 1980.

32. John Eisenberg and Arnold Rosoff, "Physician Responsibility for the Cost of Unnecessary Medical Services," *New England Journal of Medicine* vol. 299 no. 2 (July 13, 1978): 76-80.

33. Rosemary Stevens, *American Medicine and the Public Interest* (New Haven: Yale University Press, 1971), p. 423.

34. Called TOPPE for Training of Physicians for Patient Education, the group is composed of representatives from the Bureau of Health Manpower, the Bureau of Health Education, the National Cancer Institute, the National Heart, Lung, and Blood Institutes, the Bureau of Drugs, the National Library of Medicine, and some consulting physicians in family practice.

35. Ivan Illich, *Medical Nemesis: The Expropriation of Health* (London: Calder and Boyars, 1975).

36. John Knowles, "The Responsibility of the Individual," *Doing Better and Feeling Worse*, ed. John Knowles, (New York: Norton, 1977), pp. 57-80.

37. Robert Veatch "Voluntary Risks to Health," *J.A.M.A.* vol. 243 no. 1 (January 4 1980): 50-55.

38. Wesley B. Mason, et al., "Why People are Hospitalized," *Medical Care* vol. 18 no. 2 (February 1980): 147-63.

39. Knowles, "The Responsibility of the Individual", p. 80.

40. "Medicine Threatened, Economist Warns," *American Medical News* (April 14, 1979).

41. Avedis Donabedien, "Issues in National Health Insurance," *A.J.P.H.* 66 (April 1976): 345-50.

42. Margaret Jay, wife of the former British Ambassador to the U.S. has called the NHS "One of the greatest achievements in contemporary British life." *Medical World News*, (August 7, 1978) p. 87.

43. "Tory Plan for NHS Reduces Overseers, Keeps Private Beds," *Medical World News*, (January 21, 1980) p. 22 and (June 9, 1980) p. 20.

44. David Mechanic, *Medical Sociology* (New York: Free Press, 1968), p. 363f.

45. Lester Breslow, "A Positive Strategy for the Nation's Health," *J.A.M.A.* vol. 242 no. 19 (November 9, 1979): 2093-95.

46. The Mexican medical schools require a minimum of one year of service from their graduates in an underserved area before conferring the final degree or *Acta*. Most of the medical graduates with whom I have talked have agreed that the experience was worthwhile and they enjoyed it; this includes American graduates from Mexican medical schools.

47. *Opinions and Reports of the Judicial Council* (Chicago: American Medical Association, 1971), pp. vii, 56-63. Unfortunately, the exposition of this principle contained in pages 56-63 deals only briefly and superficially with social responsibilities while the bulk of the discussion concerns the physician and advertising, physician relationships with the mass media, and other matters of etiquette. The intent of the Principle which I quoted seems clear enough but this intent seems almost ignored. What happened to those "honored ideals"?

CHAPTER 9

1. Mohammed Hassar and Michael Weintraub, "Uninformed Consent and the Wealthy Volunteer," *Clinical Pharmacology*, vol. 20 no. 4 (October 1976):379-86.

2. J. Bergler, E. Freis, M. Metcalfe, and A. Pennington, "Informed Consent: How Much does the Patient Understand?" *Clinical Pharmacology* vol. 27, no. 4 (April 1980):435-40.

3. Robert Veatch and Sharmon Sollitto, "Human Experimentation—The Ethical Questions Persist," *Hastings Center Report*, vol. 3 no. 3 (June 1973):1-3.

4. "Statement of Principles" of the American Society for Clinical Pharmacology and Therapeutics.

5. American Academy of Pediatrics Committee on Drugs, *Guidelines for the Ethical Conduct of Studies to Evaluate Drugs in Pediatric Populations, see Pediatrics* vol. 60, no. 1 (July 1977):91-101.

6. Sollitto and Veatch, "Human Experimentation, p. 3.

7. Bradford Gray, "An Assessment of Institutional Review Committees in Human Experimentation," *Medical Care* vol. 13, no. 4 (April 1975):318-328.

8. Louis Lasagna, *The Conflict of Interest between Physician as Therapist and as Experimenter* (Philadelphia: Society for Health and Human Values, 1975).

9. Otto Guttentag, "Ethical Problems in Human Experimentation," *Ethical Issues in Medicine*, ed. E. Fuller Torrey (Boston: Little, Brown, 1968), pp. 195-226.

10. James Childress, "Compensating Injured Research Subjects," *Hastings Center Report* vol. 6, no. 6 (December 1976):21-27.

11. Erik Erikson, "The Golden Rule and the Cycle of Life," *Hippocrates Revisited*, Roger Bulger, ed. (New York: Medcom, 1973), pp. 181-92.

12. *Proceedings of the National Symposium on Patients' Rights in Health Care*, U.S. Department of HEW, Washington, D.C. 1976, pp. 44-47.

13. Ibid, p. 41.

14. Ibid, p. 47.

15. Robert Chiles, "The Rights of Patients," *New England Journal of Medicine* vol. 277 no. 8 (August 24, 1967):409-411.

16. Paul Tillich, *The Protestant Era*, James Adams, ed. (Chicago: University of Chicago Press, 1948), p. 115.

CHAPTER 10

1. G. Vaillant et al., "Physicians' Use of Mood-Altering Drugs: A 20-Year Follow-up Report," *New England Journal of Medicine* vol. 282, no. 7 (February 12, 1970):365-70.

2. R. Little, "Hazards of Drug Dependency Among Physicians," *J.A.M.A.* vol. 218 no. 10 (December 6, 1971):1533-35.

3. S. Benson and M. Lipp, "Physician Use of Marijuana, Alcohol, and Tabacco," *American Journal of Psychiatry*, vol. 129, no. 5 (November 1972):612-16; H. R. Lewis and M. E. Lewis, *The Medical Offenders* (New York: Simon and Schuster, 1970), chapters 12 and 19.

4. P. Stolley et al., "Drug Prescribing and Use in an American Community," *Annals of Internal Medicine* vol. 76, no. 4 (April 1972):537-540.

5. H. F. Dowling, "How Do Practicing Physicians Use New Drugs?" *J.A.M.A.* vol. 185, no. 4 (July 27 1963):233-36; P. V. J. Macaroag et al., "A Study of Hospital Staff Attitudes Concerning the Comparative Merits of Antibiotics," *Clinical Pharmacology and Therapeutics* vol. 12, no. 1 (January 1971):1-12; A. Roberts and J. Visconti, "The Rational and Irrational Use of Systemic Antimicrobial Drugs," *American Journal of Hospital Pharmacy* vol. 29, no. 10 (October 1972):828-34; and D. Dunlop, "Abuse of Drugs by the Public and by Doctors," *Medical Times* vol. 100, no. 1 (January 1972):285-93.

6. Macaroag et al., "A Study of Hospital Staff...."

7. Mary Castle et al., "Antibiotic Use at Duke University Medical Center," *J.A.M.A.* Vol. 237, no. 26 (June 27, 1977):2819-22.

8. Wayne Ray et al., "Prescribing of Tetracycline to Children Less than Eight Years Old," *J.A.M.A.* vol. 237, no. 19 (May 9, 1977):2069-74.

9. Department of Health, Education, and Welfare, *The Task Force on Prescription Drugs*, Final Report (Washington: U.S. Government Printing Office, 1968).

10. M.O. Kepler, "The Cough Syrup Jungle," *American Practitioner* vol. 12, no. 9 (September 1961):681-84.

11. Valium continues to be the most widely prescribed drug in the United States. Clearly worried by the adverse publicity the abuse and misuse this drug inspired, the chairman of the board of Roche Laboratories (the manufacturer) and the medical director appeared on national television to explain that the drug wasn't abused much and rarely misused. It sounded very defensive and lacked credibility.

12. H. Faigel, "The Marketing of Fixed Combination Pharmaceuticals," *Clinical Pediatrics* vol. 9, no. 1 (January 1970):1-2.

13. R. Dugg et al., "Use of Utilization Review to Assess the Quality of Pediatric Inpatient Care," *Pediatrics* vol. 49, no. 2 (February 1972):169-76.

14. E. Pellegrino, "Meddlesome Medicine and Rational Therapeutics," *Drug Intelligence and Clinical Pharmacy* 9 (September 1975):480-84.

15. M.O. Kepler, "The Abuse of Drug Abuse," *Clinical Pediatrics* vol. 11, no. 7 (July 1972):386-94.

16. E. Lipinski, "Motivation in Drug Abuse," *J.A.M.A.* vol. 219, no. 2 (January 10, 1977):171-75.

17. Ecclus. 30:4.

CHAPTER 11

1. Paul C. Holinger, Donald A. Tubesing, Edward A. Lichter, and Granger E. Westberg, The holistic health center project, *Medical Care* vol. 15 no. 3 (March 1977):217-27. Professor Westberg is also the author of a book entitled *Minister and Doctor Meet* published by Harper and Row in 1958 describing the common goal of the physician and clergy in a hospital setting. He is a pioneer and an outstanding authority in this field.

2. *Opinions and Reports of the Judicial Council of the AMA* (Chicago: American Medical Association, 1971) p. 47f.

3. Allen J. Brands, "Treating Ambulatory Patients: New Roles for Pharmacists," *U.S. Pharmacist* vol. 2 no. 8 (September 1977): 70-74.

4. *Together: A Casebook of Joint Practices in Primary Care*, (Chicago: National Joint Practice Commission, 1977).

5. Lynda Boyer, Corinne Kirchner, and David Lee, "A Student-run Course in Interprofessional Relations," *J. Medical Education* 52 (March 1977): 183-89.

6. One such program is called Human Dimensions in Medical Education and is offered four or more times a year. Many of the concepts used in these seminars originated in the writings of Carl R. Rogers. Further information can be obtained from the Center for Studies of the Person, 1125 Torrey Pines Road, La Jolla, California 92037.

CHAPTER 12

1. The lab coat was borrowed from the German medical schools in which it was associated with the strong foundation of biological science and therefore became the mantle of a scientist and researcher. In many medical institutions the lab coat in this country signifies a faculty person and/or a member of the senior attending staff. In recent years the lab coat has become a symbol of upward mobility as it appears in nursing education circles, among social workers, and even occasionally in a laboratory.

2. See *TIME* for May 20, 1974, p. 62. The article headed "Cutthroat Premeds" stressed the fierce competition associated with the ratio of three applicants for every first-year slot in American medical schools. The fight for a high GPA is so intensive, the article stated, that learning was secondary. Sabotage of the work of other premedical students was documented plus such trickery as stealing scarce reserve books which were required reading. Cheating was common, and there was no spirit of cooperation among premeds but rather one of savage competiton. The article concluded that "cutthroat medical students could well make cutthroat physicians." The NBC's "Weekend Report" for August 6, 1977 reflected the *TIME* findings plus an exposé concerning sums of money paid to certain medical schools which favorably influenced admission of a given student and a scandal involving thousands of dollars paid by anxious parents to Pennsylvania legislators who would use their influence on state supported schools for favored admissions.

3. There are numerous reports in the literature documenting such qualities as authoritarianism and machiavellianism in medical students. A helpful reference source is the bibliography section of each issue of the *Journal of Medical Education* published monthly by the Association of American Medical Colleges, see especially the section headed "Students."

4. One medical student produced a short film depicting a typical interview between an applicant and faculty member of the admissions committee during which the thoughts of each were audible between the spoken lines. The underly-

ing theme is that the applicant tries to give the proper responses to the interviewer's questions, but it is clear that both participants realize that this is gamesmanship. As the students say, it is a matter of "psyching out" the interviewer.

5. There were always a number of such patients around the older "free dispensary" services of my student days as there are in the public ambulatory clinics today. These are the patients who have been called "worried well" since there is no evidence of organic disease to the disappointment of some students and house staff. Such patients are often quite poor with social and mental problems that have escaped notice or remedy, and they keep returning to the clinics hoping to find a resolution to the myriad somatic complaints arising from their social and mental malaise. Obviously there is a great opportunity for teaching holistic medicine in these clinics.

6. Kathryn M. Langwell, "Career Paths of First-Year Resident Physicians: A Seven-Year Study," *Journal of Medical Education* 55 (November 1980):897-905.

7. Marie R. Huag, Bebe Lavin, and Naomi Breslau, "Practice Location Preferences at Entry to Medical School," *Journal of Medical Education* 55 (April 1980): 333-38.

8. Rudolph H. Weingartner, "Selecting for Medical School," *Journal of Medical Education* 55 (November 1980):922-27.

9. T. J. Cullen et al., "Predicting First-Quarter Test Scores From the New Medical College Admission Test," *Journal of Medical Education* 55 (May 1980): 393-98.

10. Reported in *American Medical News*, June 14, 1976.

11. Earlier, the Superior Court of California and then the Supreme Court of California ruled that the University of California School of Medicine at Davis had discriminated against a white applicant named Bakke in the preferential acceptance of less-qualified minority applicants in violation of both state and federal equal protection clauses. The case was then accepted for adjudication by the United States Supreme Court at the request of the University. Two good reviews may be found in both *Time* and *Newsweek* for July 10, 1978.

12. For one commentary on the dilemma faced by admissions committees *see* Frederick J. Ramsay, "The Medical School Admission Dilemma," *J.A.M.A.* 237 (March 14, 1977):1093-94.

13. Chase Kimball, "Medical Education as a Humanizing Process," *Journal of Medical Education* 48 (January 1973):71-77.

14. Jannice Owens and Ruth Shepherd, "Coordination of Counseling Services for Medical Students," *Pulse* 1 (March 1976): 3-6. Counseling services includes faculty advisors, student advisors, and psychiatric counseling. The students also wanted counseling services to help in choosing a medical specialty and a residency program.

15. Barbara Korsch, and Edwenna Werner "The Vulnerability of the Medical Student: Posthumous Presentation of L.L. Stephens' Ideas," *Pediatrics* 57 (March 1976): 321-27.

16. M. O. Kepler, "Ethico-Religious Instruction in Medical Schools of the U.S.," *Journal of Religion and Health* 7 (July 1968): 242-53.

17. M. O. Kepler, "Medical Schools, Religion, and Human Values," *Journal of Medical Education* 43 (September 1968):984-88.

18. M. O. Kepler, "Evaluation by Two Groups of Medical Students of a Course in Medicine and Religion," *Nebraska State Medical Journal* 57 (May 1972):171-74.

19. M. O. Kepler and Harry Saslow, "Attitudinal Changes in Medical Students Taking a Course in Human Values," *Southern Medical Journal* 69 (January 1976):21-23; and M. O. Kepler, "A Study of Some Short-Term Effects Related to a Course in Human Values," *Journal of Medical Education,* 52 (February 1977): 160.

20. Louis Lasagna, "Can One Teach Medical Ethics?" *Hippocrates Revisited* ed. Roger Bulger (New York: Medcom Press, 1973), pp. 229-36.

21. Earl R. Babbie, *Science and Morality in Medicine* (Berkeley: University of California Press, 1970).

22. Robert Veatch, *Case Studies in Medical Ethics* (Cambridge: Harvard University Press, 1977).

23. Howard Brody, *Ethical Decisions in Medicine* (Boston: Little, Brown, 1976).

24. S. Sollitto and R. Veatch, "Medical Ethics Teaching," *J.A.M.A.* vol. 235 no. 10 (March 8, 1976):1030-33.

25. See the report *Human Values Teaching Programs for Health Professionals* ed. T. McElhinney (Philadelphia: Society for Health and Human Values, 1976), p. xii. The first humanities department in a school of medicine was at the Pennsylvania State University school at Hershey in 1967. Southern Illinois School of Medicine and Wright State University School of Medicine by 1976 indicated they had departments of humanities. Eastern Virginia Medical School has had a Human Values Program since its founding in 1967. This author initiated a Human Values Program at George Washington University School of Medicine in 1965 and at the University of Nebraska School of Medicine in 1967.

26. It is interesting to see what Sir William had to say about this matter of liberal reading and the books he recommended. How many of today's medical students have encountered any of these?

Bed-Side Library for Medical Students

A liberal education may be had at a very slight cost of time and money. Well filled though the day be with appointed tasks, to make the best possible use of your one or of your ten talents, rest not satisfied with this professional training, but try to get the education, if not of a scholar, at least of a gentleman. Before going to sleep read for half an hour, and in the morning have a book open on your dressing table. You will be surprised to find how much can be accomplished in the course of a year. I have put down a list of ten books which you may make close friends. There are many others; studied carefully in your student days these will help in the inner education of which I speak.

I. Old and New Testament
II. Shakespeare
III. Montaigne
IV. Plutarch's *Lives*
V. Marcus Aurelius
VI. Epictetus

VII. *Religio Medici*
VIII. *Don Quixote*
IX. Emerson
X. Oliver Wendell Holmes—*Breakfast Table Series*

The above was taken from William Osler, *Aequanimitas* (Philadelphia: Blakiston, 1932).

27. Edmund Pellegrino, *Humanism and the Physician* (Knoxville: University of Tennessee Press, 1979), p. xi.

28. Robert L. Dickman, Leonard A. Katz, Randolph E. Sarnacki, and Frank T. Schimpfhauser, "Medical Students from Natural Science and Nonscience Undergraduate Backgrounds," *J.A.M.A.*, vol. 243, no. 24 (June 27, 1980):2506-9.

29. For an excellent article on the experiences of medical students in such an assignment, *see*: Arthur W. McMahon and Miles F. Shore, "Some Psychological Reactions to Working with the Poor," *Archives of General Psychiatry* 18 (May 1968):562-68.

30. Virginia Fine and Mark Therrien, "Empathy in the Doctor-Patient Relationship: Skill Training for Medical Students," *Journal of Medical Education* 52 (September 1977):752-57.

31. *Conditions and Problems in the Nation's Nursing Homes*, Hearings before the Subcommittee on Long-term Care of the Special Committee on Aging, United States Senate, Eighty-Ninth Congress (Washington, D. C.: Government Printing Office, 1965), p. 615. It is little wonder that the AMA opposed Doctor Knowles' nomination as assistant secretary of the then Department of HEW since he was an outspoken advocate of social reform and quality medical care for all. His untimely death in 1979 was a great loss to the nation.

32. Some encouraging activity in the teaching of cost containment was documented in a recent issue of the *Journal of Medical Education*. The entire issue reported efforts by various medical schools to teach the importance of cost control and some ways this could be accomplished such as utilization review of medical facilities and diagnostic procedures. See *Journal of Medical Education* vol. 54 no. 11 (November 1979).

33. Kelly West, "The Case Against Teaching," *Journal of Medical Education* 41 (August 1966):766-71.

CHAPTER 13

1. The definition of the word "cosmos" is illuminating in this context. Several standard dictionaries state that cosmos refers to the universe as "ordered, harmonious, and whole" or means any ordered system as opposed to chaos. The word itself derives from the Greek word *kosmos*, meaning order, universe, or world.

2. Ralph H. Major, *A History of Medicine* (Springfield: Thomas, 1954), p. 125.

3. A P. d'Entrèves, *Natural Law* (London: Hutchinson, 1951), p. 20.

4. Ibid, pp. 40-41.

5. Ibid, p. 29.

6. Paul Tillich, *Systematic Theology*, vol. 3 (Chicago: The University of Chicago Press, 1963). pp. 275-82.

7. Van Renssalaer Potter, *Bioethics: Bridge to the Future* (Englewood Cliffs: Prentice-Hall, 1971).

8. For a frightening but well-supported account of what can happen if we continue with our present and largely unrestricted policies in regard to our biosphere, *see* Jorgen Randers, "Global Limitations and Human Responsibility," *To Create a Better Future*, ed. Kenneth Vaux (New York: Friendship Press, 1972).

9. C. H. Waddington, *The Ethical Animal* (Chicago: Phoenix, 1967), pp. 28-29.

10. *Newsweek*, (October 16, 1978) p. 118. This is a good review of the current thinking of some of the authorities in the field of sociobiology.

11. These trends are stated in virtually every standard work on public health. For a discussion of this topic, *see* Eric J. Cassell, *The Healer's Art* (Philadelphia: J. B. Lippincott, 1976), pp. 74-75.

12. d'Entrèves, *Natural Law*, pp. 48-63.

13. René Dubos and Barbara Ward, *Only One Earth* (New York: W. W. Norton, 1972), p. 217.

BIBLIOGRAPHY

A.M.A. Quick Reference Guide to policies, positions and statements of the American Medical Association in regard to key health issues. Chicago: American Medical Association, 1976.

Annals of the American Academy of Political and Social Science. The Nation's Health: Some Issues, January 1972.

Annals of the New York Academy of Sciences. Home Medications and the Public Welfare. Vol. 122, pp. 807-1024. Report of a conference dealing with various aspects of self-health care with special attention to self-medication. July 19, 1965.

Augenstein, Leroy G. *Come, Let Us Play God.* New York: Harper and Row, 1969.

Bliss, Ann A. and Cohen, Eva D., eds. *The New Health Professionals.* Germantown: Aspen, 1977.

Brattgard, Helge. *God's Stewards: A Theological Study of the Principles and Practices of Stewardship.* Translated by Gene J. Lund. Minneapolis: Augsburg, 1963.

Burns, Chester R. *Legacies in Ethics and Medicine.* New York: Science History Publications, 1977.

———. *Legacies in Law and Medicine.* New York: Science History Publications, 1977.

Burrow, James G. *A.M.A. Voice of American Medicine.* Baltimore: Johns Hopkins Press, 1963.

———. *Organized Medicine in the Progressive Era: The Move Toward Monopoly.* Baltimore: Johns Hopkins Press, 1977.

Cabot, R. and Dicks, R. *The Art of Ministering to the Sick.* New York: Macmillan, 1936.

Cassell, Eric J. *The Healer's Art: A New Approach to the Doctor-Patient Relationship.* Philadelphia: J. B. Lippincott, 1976.

Clendening, Logan. *Source Book of Medical History.* New York: Dover, 1960.

Clouser, K. Danner. *Teaching Bioethics: Strategies, Problems, and Resources.* Hastings-on-Hudson: The Hastings Center, 1980.

Cutler, Donald R., ed. *Updating Life and Death.* Boston: Beacon Press, 1969.

Dawson, George G. *Healing: Pagan and Christian.* New York: Macmillan, 1935.

Dedek, John F. *Contemporary Medical Ethics.* New York: Sheed and Ward, 1975.

d'Entrèves, Alexander P. *Natural Law: An Introduction to Legal Philosophy.* London: Hutchinson University Library, 1951.

Dunham, Chester F. *Christianity in a World of Science.* New York: Macmillan, 1930.

Evans, Lester J. *The Crisis in Medical Education.* Ann Arbor: University of Michigan Press, 1964.

Fletcher, Joseph. *The Ethics of Genetic Control: Ending Reproductive Roulette*. Garden City: Anchor Books, 1974.

———. *Humanhood: Essays in Biomedical Ethics*. Buffalo: Prometheus, 1979.

———. *Morals and Medicine*. Boston: Beacon Press, 1960.

Fostering Ethical Values During the Education of Health Professionals. Philadelphia: Society for Health and Human Values, 1974.

Frazier, Claude. *Is It Moral to Modify Man?* Springfield: Charles C. Thomas, 1973.

Freeman, Howard A. et al. *Handbook of Medical Sociology*. Englewood Cliffs: Prentice-Hall, 1963.

Garlick, Phyllis L. *Man's Search for Health: A Study in the Interrelation of Religion and Medicine*. London: Highway Press, 1952.

Gorovitz, Samuel et al., eds. *Moral Problems in Medicine*. Englewood Cliffs: Prentice-Hall, 1976.

Greenberg, Selig. *The Quality of Mercy: A Report on the Critical Condition of Hospital and Medical Care in America*. New York: Atheneum, 1971.

Harmer, Ruth M. *American Medical Avarice*. New York: Abelard Schuman, 1975.

Heilbroner, Robert L. *The Worldly Philosophers: The Lives, Times and Ideas of the Great Economic Thinkers*. New York: Simon and Schuster, 1967.

Herzog, Elizabeth. *About the Poor: Some Facts and Some Fictions*. U.S. Department of HEW, Children's Bureau, Washington: U.S. Government Printing Office, 1967.

Hospers, John. *Human Conduct: An Introduction to the Problems of Ethics*. New York: Harcourt Brace Jovanovich, 1961.

Human Values Teaching Programs for Health Professionals. Philadelphia: Society for Health and Human Values, 1976. An update was due in 1980.

Hunt, Robert and Arras, John, eds. *Ethical Issues in Modern Medicine*. Palo Alto: Mayfield Publishing Company, 1977.

Illich, Ivan. *Medical Nemesis: The Expropriation of Health*. New York: Pantheon Books, 1976.

Irelan, Lola M., ed. *Low-Income Life Styles*. U. S. Department of H.E.W., Washington: U. S. Government Printing Office, 1966.

Jakobovits, Immanuel. *Jewish Medical Ethics*. New York: Bloch, 1975.

Johnson, Ernest F., ed. *Patterns of Ethics in America Today*. New York: Crowell-Collier, 1962.

The Journal of Medical Education. 54:11 (November 1979) Virtually the entire issue is devoted to the teaching of cost containment in U. S. medical schools.

Kelly, Gerald A. *Medico-Moral Problems*. St. Louis: Catholic Hospital Association, 1958.

Kieffer, George H. *Bioethics: A Textbook of Issues*. Reading: Addison-Wesley Publishing Co., 1979.

Knowles, John H., ed. *Doing Better and Feeling Worse*. New York: Norton, 1977.

———. *Views of Medical Education and Medical Care*. Cambridge: Harvard University Press, 1968.

Kosa, John, ed. *Poverty and Health*. Cambridge: Harvard University Press, 1975.

Lappé, Marc and Morrison, Robert S., eds. "Ethical and Scientific Issues Posed by Human Uses of Molecular Genetics." *Annals of the New York Academy of Sciences*, Vol 265, 1971.

Lapsley, James N. *Salvation and Health: The Interlocking Processes of Life.* Philadelphia: Westminster, 1972.

Lasagna, Louis C. *The Doctors' Dilemmas.* New York: Harper and Row, 1962.

Lipkin, Mack Jr. and Rowley, Peter T., eds. *Genetic Responsibility: On Choosing Our Children's Genes.* New York: Plenum Press, 1974.

Major, Ralph. *A History of Medicine* (Two volumes). Springfield: Thomas, 1954.

Margotta, Roberto. *The Story of Medicine.* New York: Golden Press, 1967.

McKeown, Thomas and Lowe, Charles R. *An Introduction to Social Medicine.* Oxford: Blackwell Scientific Publications, 1974.

Mechanic, David. *Medical Sociology: A Selective View.* New York: The Free Press, 1968.

"Medical Ethics and Social Change", *The Annals of the American Academy of Political and Social Science.* 437: (May 1978).

Medical School Admission Requirements. 30th ed. Washington, D.C.: Association of American Medical Colleges, 1980.

Mendelson, Mary A. *Tender Loving Greed: How the Incredibly Lucrative Nursing Home Industry is Exploiting America's Old People and Defrauding Us All.* New York: Vantage, 1975.

Moore, Wilbert E. *The Professions: Roles and Rules.* New York: Russell Sage Foundation, 1970.

Moss, Frank E. and Halamandaris, Val J. *Too Old Too Sick Too Bad.* Germantown: Aspen, 1977.

Nelson, James B. *Human Medicine: Ethical Perspectives on New Medical Issues.* Minneapolis: Augsburg Publishing Company, 1973.

Noonan, John P. *General and Special Ethics.* Chicago: Loyola University Press, 1947.

Pellegrino, Edmund D. *Humanism and the Physician.* Knoxville: University of Tennessee Press, 1979.

Pike, James A. *Doing the Truth: A Summary of Christian Ethics.* Garden City: Doubleday, 1955.

The Place of Value Systems in Medical Education. New York: The Academy of Religion and Mental Health.

Potter, Van Rensselaer. *Bioethics: Bridge to the Future.* Englewood Cliffs: Prentice-Hall, 1971.

Reiser, Stanley J. et al. *Ethics in Medicine: Historical Perspectives and Contemporary Concerns.* Cambridge: MIT Press, 1977.

Robinson, Victor. *The Story of Medicine.* New York: Tudor, 1931.

Sahakian, William S. *Ethics: An Introduction to Theories and Problems.* New York: Harper and Row, 1974.

Sanders, Marion K., ed. *The Crisis in American Medicine.* New York: Harper and Brothers, 1961.

Shinn, Roger L. *Tangled World.* New York: Charles Scribner's Sons, 1965.

Sperry, Willard. *The Ethical Basis of Medical Practice.* New York: Hoeber, 1950.

Stevens, Robert B. and Stevens, Rosemary. *Welfare Medicine in America: A Case Study of Medicaid.* New York: Free Press, 1974.

Stevens, Rosemary. *American Medicine and the Public Interest.* New Haven: Yale University Press, 1971.

———— et al. *The Alien Doctors: Foreign Medical Graduates in American Hospitals.* New York: John Wiley and Sons, 1978.

Szasz, Thomas S. *The Theology of Medicine: The Political-Philosophical Foundation of Medical Ethics.* New York: Harper and Row, 1977.

Tancredi, Laurence R., ed. *Ethics of Health Care.* Washington: National Academy of Science, 1971.

Tomlin, Eric W. F. *The Western Philosophers; An Introduction.* New York: Harper and Row, 1963.

Torrey, E. Fuller and Badgley, Robin F., eds. *Ethical Issues in Medicine: The Role of the Physician in Today's Society.* Boston: Little, Brown and Company, 1968.

Vaux, Kenneth L., ed. *Who Shall Live?: Medicine, Technology, Ethics.* Philadelphia: Fortress Press, 1970.

Veatch, Robert M. *Case Studies in Medical Ethics.* Cambridge: Harvard University Press, 1977.

———— and Branson, Roy, eds. *Ethics and Health Policy.* Cambridge: Ballinger, 1976.

———— et al. *The Teaching of Medical Ethics.* Hastings-on-Hudson: Hastings Center, 1973.

Visscher, Maurice B., ed. *Humanistic Perspectives in Medical Ethics.* Buffalo: Prometheus, 1972.

Waddams, Herbert M. *A New Introduction to Moral Theology.* London: Student Christian Movement, 1964.

Waddington, Conrad H. *The Ethical Animal.* Chicago: University of Chicago Press, 1967.

Watkin, Edward I. *The Church in Council.* London: Darton, 1961.

White, Dale, ed. *Dialogue in Medicine and Theology.* Nashville, Abingdon, 1968.

Ward, Barbara and Dubos, René. *Only One Earth: The Care and Maintenance of a Small Planet.* New York: W. W. Norton, 1972.

Wilson, E. O. *On Human Nature.* Cambridge: Harvard University Press, 1978.

AUTHOR INDEX

Al-Ruhawi, 14
Amundsen, D. W., 14
Aquinas, Thomas, 211
Augenstein, Leroy, 87

Babbie, Earl R., 199
Bachman, Leonard, 142
Belli, Melvin, 171
Breslow, Lester, 133
Brody, Howard, 200
Burns, Chester, 20-21

Callahan, Daniel, 104
Chiles, Robert, 144
Cicero, 211
Crile, George, Jr., 47-48

Derbyshire, Robert C., 62, 109
Donabedian, Avedis, 130
Dowling, Henry, 150
Dunlop, Sir Derrick, 150
Duvalier, "Papa Doc," 85-86

Edelstein, Ludwig, 4, 5, 6, 7, 16
Enthove, Alain G., 129
Entralgo, P. L., 3
Erikson, Erik, 141

Faigel, H., 155
Fletcher, Joseph, 12, 13, 83, 87
Flexner, Abraham, 27, 107

Galen, 10, 13, 14
Guttentag, Otto, 140

Illich, Ivan, 127, 129
Israel, Isaac, 14

Kimball, Chase, 193
Knowles, John, 128, 205

Lappé, Marc, 92
Largus, Scribonius, 16
Lasagna, Louis, 150, 198-199
Levey, M., 14
Lewis, C. S., 212
Lipinski, E., 157

McCaulley, Mary, 187-188, 195
McMahon, John A., 143
Major, Ralph, 8
Maritain, Jacques, 212
Mechanic, David, 131
Moore, Wilbert E., 17

Nader, Ralph, 59

Osler, William, 201
Osmundsen, John, 95

Pellegrino, Edmund, 201-202
Percival, Thomas, 20, 21, 38, 170
Plato, 14

Potter, Van Rensselaer, 213

Sade, Robert, 104
Securis, John, 161
Self, Donnie, 103, 195
Shirkey, Harry, 163
Slater, Philip, 90
Socrates, 204
Sollitto, S., 201
Szasz, Thomas, 72

Tillich, Paul, 145, 212

Vaillant, G., 147
Van Dusen, Henry, 88
Veatch, Robert M., 200, 201
Virchow, Rudolf, 158

Waddington, C. H., 214
Weingartner, Rudolph H., 185
West, Kelly, 207
Westberg, Granger, 160

SUBJECT INDEX

abortion, 6, 96-100

adulation disease, 77, 153, 171

advocacy role, *philia* and responsibility, 76

advocacy role of the physician, 6, 19, 73-77

agape, 3, 10

allocation of scarce medical resources, 84

ambulatory surgery, 125

American Academy of Pediatrics, 137

American Board of Family Practice, 57

American Hospital Association, 141, 143

American Medical Association, 19, 24

  accreditation of nursing homes and, 34

  black medical schools and, 28

  cost of medical care and, 39-41

  Council on Medical Education, 27

  Department of Medicine and Religion, 78, 160

  doctor-patient relationship and, 42

  Drug Evaluations and, 36

  fee-splitting and, 47

  Fishbein era of, 29

  fraud and abuse in Medicaid-Medicare and, 32

  free immunizations and examinations of school children and, 33

  goals of, 26

  liberal period of, 29

  Medicaid physicians' earnings and, 46

  medical care as a right and, 31

  medical education and, 27, 30, 31

  medical malpractice and, 37

  Model Constitution and By-laws for a Medical Society, 25-26, 38

  as a monopoly, 33

  national health insurance and, 29, 33, 130

  opposition to amendments to Food and Drug Act and, 36

  Percival's *Medical Ethics* and, 38

  physician ownership of pharmacies and, 162

  physician shortage and, 28, 32, 108

  political strength of, 34-35

  prepaid health plans and, 33-34

  public health and, 33

  recommendation that teaching of medical ethics be required, 196-197

relations with the drug industry, 35
relations with the Pharmaceutical Manufacturers' Association and, 35-36
Social Security and, 33
socialized medicine and, 32, 41
tobacco industry and, 36
American Society for Clinical Pharmacology and Therapeutics, 137
amniocentesis, 92, 100
Asklepiads, 8
Asklepion, Koan, 8
Asklepios, 8
Asklepios, cult of, 8

Babylon 15
Bakke case, 189
Bachman, Leonard, 142
barriers to health care, 105-106
bioethical Creed (Potter's), 213, 249-250
bioethics, 213
  defined, 213
biofeedback, 95
biosphere, 210
  ethical conduct and, 213
birth defects, 91
Book of Common Prayer, 212
British National Health Service, 48
Blue Cross-Blue Shield, 49, 115, 125, 126

caring in medicine, 102-103, 133, 139, 141
caritas, 3
Carnegie Foundation for the Advancement of Teaching, 178
China, health rights of the group and, 100, 132

Chinese medicine, 7, 100, 132
Christ as the Great Physician, 10
Christian contributions to medical ethics, 9
Christian hospice, 10
  agape, 10
  stewardship, 10-12, 82
church clinic, 161
clergy in medicine, 159-161
  antagonism vs. collaboration with physicians and, 160
  clinical pastoral training and, 159
  counseling skills in stress and, 159
  need for, 161
clinical trials for drugs, 135
Code of Hammurabi, 15
Code of Ethics, AMA, xiv
codes of conduct, 15
comforter role of the physician, 77-82
community health centers, 115
competence, professional, 6, 7, 13, 19, 23, 53
  AMA Principles of Medical Ethics and, 56
  continuing education and, 55-56
  defined, 53-54
  educational standards for, 54-55
  medical licensure boards and, 55
  peer review need for, 57
  remedial mechanisms for lack of, 66
consanguinity, 95
consumerism, 59, 74
Coordinating Council on Medical Education, 31, 54
cost containment
  cost-sharing by patient and, 125

cost-sharing of health services by consumers, 125
health-care education and, 126
health maintenance organization, 123-124
high-risk individuals and, 128-129
individual responsibility and, 127-128
peer review and, 124
physicians and, 124, 130
self-health care and, 129
unnecessary surgery and, 124

Declaration of Geneva, 7, 243
disciplinary mechanisms, 60
disciplinary tradition of medicine, 23, 46, 56
disease
    as disharmony, 11
    as disharmony with nature, 211
    due to failure of right conduct, 212
disease incidence in poverty areas, 114
divine economy, 11
drug abuse
    by physicians, 146-147
    physicians as experts and, 146
    ways in which physicians may increase problems and, 147-150
drug advertising, 151, 154
drug misuse
    at Johns Hopkins Hospital and Duke University Medical Center, 151
    by physicians, 151-152
drug prescribing, 148-151
    ethical aspects, 155
    excessive use of psychoactive drugs and, 148-149

inadequate knowledge of by physicians and, 150-152
inappropriate use of antibiotics and, 150-152
of irrational drugs, 155-156
peer review and, 156
regulatory agencies and, 156
to please patients, 153-154

East Coast Migrant Health Project, 115
Eastern Virginia Medical School, 186, 195
ecological balances, 213
elderly
    health care needs of, 115
    the way we care for, 90
empires, Byzantine and Islamic, 13
ethical behavior
    development of, 214
    social and genetic factors in, 214
ethical wheel, 23, 43, 69
ethico-religious instruction, 197
ethics, distinguished from morals and etiquette, xiii
ethics of health cost containment, 124-130
euthanasia, 86-90
    and the Nazis, 89
experimentation on humans, 135-141
    compensation for injured subjects and, 139
    conflicts of interest and, 140
    ethics committees and, 139
    Golden Rule and, 141
    medical schools and, 140-141
    philial partnership and, 140
    risk/benefit ratio and, 139
    use of children, prisoners, the disadvantaged and, 137-138

Fall of Man, 215
family medicine training programs, 110-112
Federal Food and Drug Administration, 150-153
fee-for-service method of providing health care, 45, 47, 50, 120
Fishbein, Morris, 29-30
Flexner Report, 27-28
Food and Drug Act, Harris-Kefauver Amendments to, 152
foreign medical graduates, 108-110
free-market system of medical care, 113
Fry, Elizabeth, 164

General Motors and medical costs, 40
genetic disease, 91
"genetic engineering," 95, 215
genetic screening, 91-100
"genetic twilight," 92-93
Golden Rule in medicine, 141, 144
Graduate Medical Education National Advisory Committee, 112-113, 183
Greek medicine as "pagan," 10
guild tradition in medicine, 19, 22

health, wholeness, and salvation, 212
health care as a right, 103-105
health care insurance, 113
Health Manpower Act of 1976, 109
health manpower problems, 106-113
Health Maintenance Organization, 125-126
Health Systems Agency, 40

Hellenic period, 6
Hippocrates, 4-9
Hippocratic Corpus, 7, 211
Hippocratic legacy, 46, 51, 69, 85, 97, 123, 124, 133, 144, 177, 210, 213
defined, xviii
Hippocratic Oath, 4-7
acceptance by early Christians, 9
advocacy role in, 6
brotherhood of physicians in, 6, 169
philia, implied in, 6
professional competence and, 6
text of, 5
holistic healing, 72
hospital chaplain, 160, 161
human behavior as genetically determined, 215
humanhood, criteria for, 83-84
humanhood and genetic disease, 97
humanism, Greek, 6
Humanitas, 16
human pollution, 218
human values in medicine program, 195

Imhotep, 4
impaired physician, 56-57
informed consent, 135-136
inter-professional relationships, 158

Jehovah's Witnesses, 74, 99
Jews, and one source of healing, 9
Judaic contributions to medical ethics, 9
Justinian emperor, 10

Koan school of medicine, 8

Lab coat mentality, 179, 183
living wills, 90, 241-242

McMahon, John A., 143
Marcus brothers, 67
marketplace medicine, 45, 47, 49
and the poor, 50-52
martyr syndrome in physicians, 171
"Medicaid mills," 46, 51, 155
medical administration's interaction with physicians, 167-169
medical education
as a dehumanizing process, 193
Hippocratic Oath and, 27
as a humanizing process, 193
role of comforter for the physician and, 81
medical ethics, defined, xiii
medical college admission assessment program , 186-187
Medical College Admission Test, 179, 186-187
medical educators, study of, 199
medical ethics, teaching of, 197-201
medicalization of life, 127, 129
medical profession's need to reform, 219
medical school admissions, 184-192
Bakke case and, 189
bribes and contributions to obtain, 180
eventual practice location and, 189
fierce competition and, 180, 184
high MCAT and GPA scores and, 179-180

minority applicants and, 189-190
need for noncognitive assessment and, 186-188
personality testing and, 186
stress and, 180
suggestions for improvement of, 185
training in humanistics and, 188
typical applicant for, 180
medical schools
corporate ethics of, 208
curriculum muddle and, 196-203
ethical obligation to select faculty, 203
freedom to admit whom they wish, 191
influence on basic attitudes of medical students, 203
public accountability and, 178
responsibility and autonomy in selecting applicants, 191
teaching of medical ethics and, 197-198
Medicare-Medicaid programs, 116-121
abuse of by health care providers, 46, 119-120
costs of, 118
fee-for-service and abuse of, 20
near financial collapse of, 131
nursing homes and, 121
overutilization of hospitals in, 119
Patients' Bill of Rights and, 143
reasons for limited success of, 219
Senator Frank E. Moss and, 120
utilization of health services and, 117

medicine
  as politics on a small scale 158
  self-healing needed of, 123
  service tradition of, 15, 18, 19,
    51
  as a social science, 158
  state regulation of, 13
"Medicine, Religion, and Healing,"
  197
Mexican medical schools, and Social service, 134
mid-level practitioner, 165
migrant workers, health care of,
  114
Minneapolis Multiphasic Personality Inventory, 204

national health centers, 115
national health insurance, 130
National Health Service (British),
  131-132
natural law, 210-213
natural rights theory, 217-218
need for ethical leaning, 214
neighborhood health centers, 115
Nork, John, 62-64, 66
Nuremberg Code, 137
nurse practitioner, 165-166
nursing profession, 164-167
  beginnings in early Christianity,
    164
  competition between the medi-
    cal profession and, 166
  expansion of after World War II,
    165
  Hippocratic legacy and philia in,
    166
  National Joint Practice Com-
    mission, 167
  secular nursing orders, 164
  shortage of nurses in, 165

omniscient wonder worker sickness in physicians, 171

patient education, 126-127
Patients' Bill of Rights, 74, 141-
  143, 223-226
patient trust, 76-77
peer review
  in antiquity, 12-13
  cost containment and, 124
Percival's Code of Ethics (1803),
  170
Percival's Medical Ethics, 38
Personality Orientation Inventory,
  186
personality types, 187
pharmacist
  duty to check physicians' pre-
    scriptions and, 162
  expanded role of, 163
  patient care and, 163-164
pharmacy profession, 161-164
philia
  as agape or caritas, 3
  as brotherly love, xv
  euthanasia and, 88
  failure to practice as the basic
    disorder of man, 217
  in the Hippocratic Oath, 6
  as key factor in humanization or
    dehumanization of students,
    193
  Medicare-Medicaid programs
    and, 123
  nursing homes and, 81
  stewardship and, 86
  toward the disadvantages, 51
philiotekne, 14
physician extenders, 108
physicians
  as an agent of God, 71

desirable qualities of, 13, 186
ego gratification needs and, 171
as exemplars, 157
humility in, 72
interaction with clergy and, 158
interviewing skills and, 205
maldistribution and GMENAC report, 112
and nursing homes, 79-81
paternalism in, 73
as priest, 70-73
as a professional, 19
self-regulation, 13
shortage and maldistribution of, 106-107
shortage in South Viet Nam, 110
social responsibilities of, 132-134
surplus by 1990, 112
unaware of their own motives, 175
physis, 211
PKU disease, 95
placebo, use of in clinical trials, 138
preventive health care in marketplace medicine, 49-50
primary-care physicians, 110, 165
profession
    characteristics of, 17
    meaning of, 16-17
professional person, 17
    guild tradition and, 19
Professional Standards Review Organization (PSROs), 46, 122, 123, 156
Pythagoreans, 5, 6

Quality Assessment Program, 58
quality of health care, 58-60

quality of life, 86
    growing judicial support for, 99
    and stewardship, 82, 84

"recombinant DNA," 215
responsibility, tradition in medicine, 23
responsibility and autonomy of a professional person, 17-19, 191
"right-to-death" legislation, 89
rights
    group, 98, 100-101, 132
    of patients, 144
right to health care, 103-105

salaried physician, satisfaction of, 48-49
self-euthanasia, 89
service tradition in medicine, 15, 18, 19, 51, 108, 210
sickle cell screening, 95
situation ethics, 12-13, 84, 176
social medicine
    limited success of, 219
    teaching aspects of, 206-207
socialized medicine, 131-132
    attitudes of medical faculty toward, 199
Social Security Administration, 117
sociobiologist, 95
Sociobiology, 214
    selfish genes and, 214
stewardship, 10-12, 113, 213, 218
stewardship role of the physician, 82-101
Stoicism, 6, 211, 217
Study on Surgical Services in the United States, 37

Surgeon General's report on smoking and cancer, 36
surgery
  second opinions for, 37, 48
  unnecessary, 37, 124
surgical rates under national health services, 48

Thatcher, Margaret, 131
Theodosius, emperor, 10
"Toilet Assumption," 90
truth-telling and the physician, 75
two Great Commandments, 9, 81, 217

Uniform Anatomical Gift Act, 90
United Mine Workers, 114

U.S. Congress, 115
U.S. Department of Health, Education, and Welfare's *The Task Force on Prescription Drugs* (1968), 151
U.S. Department of Health and Human Services, 116
U.S. Senate's Special Committee on Aging, 79

World Health Organization, definition of health, 132
wrongful life, 99-100

Yale Law Review article on the AMA, 44

About the Author

M. Oliver Kepler received his bachelor of arts and medical degrees from Syracuse University and a master of arts degree from George Washington University. He served in Alaska and Guatemala as a medical missionary and during the Vietnam war he was a volunteer physician for a children's plastic surgery hospital in Saigon. His academic experience includes full-time faculty appointments at the University of Nebraska School of Medicine, the Baylor School of Medicine, the Eastern Virginia Medical School; Dr. Kepler also held dual appointments in medicine and religion at George Washington University. His clinical experience has been in general practice, pediatrics, industrial medicine, public health, and care of the mentally retarded. He has published many articles dealing with the clinical and social aspects of medicine. He is a diplomate of the American Board of Pediatrics, the National Board of Medical Examiners, the American Board of Family Practice, and is a fellow of the American Society for Clinical Pharmacology and Therapeutics. Currently he is the medical director of a primary care medical clinic in New Mexico.